Communication in the Age of the COVID-19 Pandemic

Communication in the Age of the COVID-19 Pandemic

Edited by
Theresa MacNeil-Kelly

LEXINGTON BOOKS
Lanham • Boulder • New York • London

Published by Lexington Books
An imprint of The Rowman & Littlefield Publishing Group, Inc.
4501 Forbes Boulevard, Suite 200, Lanham, Maryland 20706
www.rowman.com

6 Tinworth Street, London SE11 5AL, United Kingdom

Copyright © 2021 The Rowman & Littlefield Publishing Group, Inc.

All rights reserved. No part of this book may be reproduced in any form or by any electronic or mechanical means, including information storage and retrieval systems, without written permission from the publisher, except by a reviewer who may quote passages in a review.

British Library Cataloguing in Publication Information Available

Library of Congress Cataloging-in-Publication Data

Names: MacNeil-Kelly, Theresa, 1982- editor.
Title: Communication in the age of the COVID-19 Pandemic / edited by Theresa MacNeil-Kelly.
Description: Lanham : Lexington Books, 2021. | Includes bibliographical references and index. | Summary: "Communication in the Age of the COVID-19 Pandemic centers around changes in communication as a byproduct of the COVID-19 pandemic. Specific contexts include changes in our intimate relationships and changes in how media outlets communicate to audiences"— Provided by publisher.
Identifiers: LCCN 2021030859 | ISBN 9781793639912 (cloth) | ISBN 9781793639936 (paper) | ISBN 9781793639929 (epub)
Subjects: LCSH: COVID-19 Pandemic, 2020- , in mass media. | COVID-19 Pandemic, 2020—Influence. | Communication—History—21st century. | LCGFT: Essays.
Classification: LCC P96.C69 C66 2021 | DDC 302.209/052—dc23
LC record available at https://lccn.loc.gov/2021030859

For my department colleagues—thank you for an amazing journey.

Contents

Foreword   ix
Alex Ortiz

Acknowledgments   xi

Introduction   xiii
Theresa MacNeil-Kelly

PART I: INTIMATE COMMUNICATION   1

1 Right or Wrong? An Analysis of In-law Communication during the COVID-19 Crisis   3
Cara T. Mackie

2 Talking Myself off a Ledge: Navigating Identity during COVID-19 Quarantine   19
Pamela Dykes

PART II: MASS COMMUNICATION   33

3 Sports Diplomacy in the Age of the COVID-19 Pandemic   35
Katherine Loh

4 Agenda Setting: A Thematic Analysis of *The New York Times* COVID-19 Coverage   49
Theresa MacNeil-Kelly

5 #Kidstogether: How Nickelodeon Framed Entertainment-Education Messages during the COVID-19 Pandemic   63
Jobia Keys

Index   79

About the Authors   85

Foreword
Alex Ortiz

The COVID-19 pandemic upended the world community beginning in 2020 and its final story remains far from being told. To be sure, much is known already—the disease's global death toll receives constant and unrelenting updates on the news. The daily figures represent individuals, families, and communities who have had loved ones taken away far too soon; many more will have recovered but may deal with the disease's long-lasting consequences for years to come.

Despite this ongoing coverage, much less treatment has been given to understanding the pandemic's broader role in less talked about aspects of our lives, such as its impact on family dynamics, interpersonal relationships, and what our children see on television. The writers of this book address this gap by reflecting upon the myriad ways the health crisis has affected individuals and broader society.

The text begins with an inward investigation of the role of the virus on intrapersonal and interpersonal relationships. Cara Mackie discusses the challenges of family communication efforts among members who had different perspectives of dealing with the crisis. The author provides rich detail from her personal experiences to better understand how families negotiated these differences. Pamela Dykes extends this conversation by employing an autoethnographic approach to describe navigating identity as a caregiver and Black woman during dual health and racial pandemics.

Other stories in this book turn to the discussion of media and COVID-19. Katherine Loh provides a case study analysis of Sports Diplomats' social media use during the pandemic to better understand how strategic communication reflected their role as representatives of their sport. A contribution by Theresa MacNeil-Kelly uses agenda-setting theory to analyze the *New York Times* coverage of COVID-19 from the initial stages when U.S. infections were low, to later coverage when the virus' devastating toll had become tragically apparent. Last, Jobia Keys explores the children's television network Nickelodeon and the different strategies it used to inform its young audience about the pandemic—a delicate balancing act that sought to avoid causing unwanted alarm.

All told, these writers provide readers with a valuable and needed perspective of the COVID-19 virus that has received little scholarly analysis to date. It will certainly add to a growing collection of research aimed at understanding such an unprecedented and historical pandemic.

Acknowledgments

A special thank you to the authors in this book for taking the time and energy to write these chapters. This book was a labor of love and certainly would not have been possible without their unique contributions and help in the compilation of the final text. The authors have known each other for several years and have remained, during this time, in the same department as both colleagues and friends. Thank you for this collaborative effort and for the support of all of the faculty in the communication department at Florida Southern College.

The authors would also like to thank Lexington Books for giving us the chance to share our research with others. We appreciate you giving us this opportunity.

Last, the authors of this book would like to collectively recognize our families who graciously encouraged us on this journey and allowed us to spend long hours writing and revising our research. Without this family support, our work could not be possible. Thank you all.

Introduction

Theresa MacNeil-Kelly

On December 31, 2019, the World Health Organization (WHO) first discovered several cases of pneumonia in Wuhan, China. These cases would eventually be known as COVID-19, a novel coronavirus (WHO 2020). On January 21, 2020, the first instance of COVID-19 was confirmed in the United States (U.S.) in Washington state, where a man in his thirties had contracted the virus from a recent trip to Wuhan (Taylor 2021). On January 30, 2020, the WHO announced an international health emergency and then on March 11, 2020, the WHO declared COVID-19 a global pandemic (WHO 2020).

There have been several negative changes and impacts of COVID-19 on our society, including financial and economic consequences, as well as declines in people's overall mental health and increases in substance abuse disorders (Panchal, Kamal and Garfield 2021, para. 1). Interpersonal communication is another area that has seen change due to COVID-19. The coronavirus pandemic has significantly altered how individuals communicate (Jones 2020, para. 1). Due to facial coverings and social distancing, people have had to find alternative means of greetings, gestures, and other nonverbal cues (para. 1). According to Jones (2020), "we're all being pushed into an online existence," and ultimately losing some of our in-person communication cues (para. 16). Moreover, within interpersonal relationships, conflict has also increased between romantic partners, friends and family members due to the effects of COVID-19 (MacNeil-Kelly 2021, 1).

Mass media has also seen considerable changes in communication as a consequence of COVID-19. According to Anwar et al. (2020) "mass media became the major source of information about the novel coronavirus . . . and significantly contributed to the COVID-19 infodemics" (1). Further, media coverage "induced fear" but also "played a worldwide role in coronavirus disease tracking," which "allowed for timely interventions by the Center for

Disease Control and Prevention (CDC) and the WHO, enabling rapid and widespread reach of public health communication" (1).

Thus, it is evident that in the interpersonal and mass media spheres, communication has played an important role during the COVID-19 pandemic. However, because the epidemic is so new, there is still much to learn about communication in these areas, and therefore this text hopes to expand upon the paucity of research within these spheres.

GOALS AND PURPOSE

A main purpose of the present text, *Communication in the Age of the COVID-19 Pandemic*, is to organize communication surrounding COVID-19 into two parts: intimate communication and mass communication, and to focus on how COVID-19 is managed and assessed in these areas. In addition, this collection takes the perspective that communication, particularly the message, is at the center of understanding communication research, a view shared by other scholars in the field (Oezel and Ting-Toomey 2013, viii).

A second main goal of this text is to explore the intersection of communication and COVID-19 within qualitative methodological perspectives. According to Denzin and Lincoln (2011), qualitative research "is a situated activity that locates the observer in the world" and "consists of a set of interpretive, material practices that make the world visible. These practices transform the world . . . qualitative researchers study things in their natural settings, attempting to make sense of, or interpret, phenomena in terms of the meanings people bring to them" (3). The *Communication in the Age of the COVID-19 Pandemic* text uses several different qualitative methodologies to try and comprehend the role of COVID-19 messages in intimate and media spheres, including autoethnography (chapters 1 and 2), case study (chapter 3), thematic (chapter 4), and framing (chapter 5) analyses. More specific details about the audience and organizational framework for the *Communication in the Age of the COVID-19 Pandemic* text are discussed in the next section.

AUDIENCE AND ORGANIZATIONAL FRAMEWORK

The intended audience for the *Communication in the Age of the COVID-19 Pandemic* text is primarily for those individuals who are interested in learning about new COVID-19 research, as it relates to communication. More specifically, this text is intended for (1) academics who will use it to complement their interests in communication or similar fields, (2) instructors who may use it to supplement their courses in communication or other parallel classes, (3) undergraduate and graduate students of the humanities, (4) practitioners who wish to use the current research to help others in their daily lives, and (5) individuals who can relate to experiences conveyed in the text. In essence, this text allows for all of these groups to gain an understanding of new COVID-19 research in disparate ways. Academics, instructors, and students can use this text to create interesting classroom discussion as well as promote new research ideas, and practitioners can use it to gain pragmatic solutions that will ultimately help patients and clients. Moreover, other nonacademic individuals may be interested in this text, simply because they can relate to the experiences shared, particularly with respect to the intimate accounts of COVID-19.

As mentioned previously, this text is organized into two parts: Part I and Part II. Part I discusses how individuals deal with intimate communication experiences related to COVID-19. Intimate situations involve personal experiences and therefore, chapter 1 and chapter 2 utilize autoethnography to address intimate communication surrounding COVID-19. Autoethnography, as a type of methodology, is merely a sophisticated version of an autobiographical account that combines personal and cultural observations, often mediated by language (Ellis and Bochner 2000, 742). Thus, in chapter 1, Mackie uses autoethnography to navigate her personal feelings with family during the COVID-19 crisis, focusing on communication with in-laws, using vignettes that highlight conflict and sensemaking to better understand how families navigate(d) the COVID-19 pandemic. According to Koerner (2007), family communication is comprised of psychological and interpersonal behavioral processes, the first of which is not readily observable, while the latter is clearly visible. Mackie is able to wonderfully navigate between these two types of interchanges in her autoethnographical account.

Another element of Part I in the *Communication in the Age of the COVID-19 Pandemic* text is Dykes' chapter 2 personal account of her intrapersonal communication and identity struggles. Similar to Mackie, Dykes also utilizes an autoethnographical approach to illustrate her experiences. Dykes takes the reader through several intimate narratives detailing her internal struggles during COVID-19, including navigating and managing her identity as a caregiver and African American woman during dual health and racial pandemics.

Part II of the *Communication in the Age of the COVID-19 Pandemic* text encompasses chapters 3–5 and discusses some important ways messages were communicated in the media during COVID-19. In chapter 3, Loh observes the sport of lacrosse and details social media messages from Lyle Thompson, who is considered lacrosse's most recognized Sports Diplomat (Loh, 2020).

Using this case study analysis, she examines communication messages and sports diplomacy in the time of the COVID-19 pandemic within the Native American community, a group that has been disproportionately impacted by COVID-19.

Using thematic analysis, in chapter 4, MacNeil-Kelly analyzes news media coverage in the United States in *The New York Times* during the months of March 2020 and April 2020 of the first wave of the COVID-19 virus spread in America. Guided by agenda-setting theory, she discusses salient topics in news coverage during these months and the impacts these topics may have on newsreaders.

Last, Keys rounds out the discussion on COVID-19 and media messages in Part II of chapter 5, with a discussion on how the media play a significant role in defining and framing health issues for the public. More specifically, she analyzes the framing of COVID-19 health messages within all COVID-19 related televised programming that Nickelodeon produced through digital streaming and on-demand cable services, and their impacts on mitigating the spread of the virus.

Taken together the succeeding chapters add to a growing body of COVID-19 research. Moreover, the *Communication in the Age of the COVID-19 Pandemic* text attempts to provide readers with a cohesive discussion of the qualitative findings of both intimate and media COVID-19 communication accounts. We encourage the reader to share this collection of research with others in their own personal and professional lives, and we genuinely hope they will find this text interesting, helpful, and beneficial.

REFERENCES

Anwar, Ayesha, Meryem Malik, Vaneeza Raees, and Anjum Anwar. 2020. "The Role of Mass Media and Public Health Communications in the COVID-19 Pandemic." *Cureus* 12, no. 9: 1–12. www.https://doi.org/10.7759/cureus.10453.

"Archived: WHO Timeline – COVID-19." 2020. April 27, 2020. https://www.who.int/news/item/27-04-2020-who-timeline---covid-19.

Denzin, Norman K. and Yvonna S. Lincoln. 2011. "Introduction." *The Handbook of Qualitative Research, Fourth Edition*, edited by Norman K. Denzin and Yvonna S. Lincoln, 3–9. Thousand Oaks, CA: Sage.

Ellis, Carolyn and Bochner, Arthur, P. 2000. "Autoethnography, Personal Narrative, Reflexivity." *The Handbook of Qualitative Research, Second Edition*, edited by Norman K. Denzin and Yvonna S. Lincoln, 733–768. Thousand Oaks, CA: Sage.

Jones, Tricia. "The Coronavirus Pandemic has Made Communication More Important than Ever." 2020. Accessed April 1, 2021. https://news.temple.edu/news/2020-09-16/coronavirus-pandemic-has-made-communication-more-important-ever.

Koerner, Ascan F. 2007. "Social Cognition in Family Communication." *Communication and Social Cognition: Theories and Methods*, edited by David R. Roskos-Ewoldsen and Jennifer L. Monahan, 197–216. Mahwah: Lawrence Erlbaum.

Loh, Katherine. 2020. "Sports Diplomacy and Conflict Framing: An Analysis of How Celebrity Athletes Influence Discourse in Race and Politics." *The Role of Conflict on the Individual and Society*, edited by Theresa MacNeil-Kelly, 87–102, Lanham: Lexington Press.

MacNeil-Kelly, Theresa. 2021. "Quarantining amidst COVID-19: An Analysis of Romantic Couple Conflict." [Manuscript in preparation], Department of Communication, Florida Southern College.

Oetzel, John G. and Stella Ting-Toomey. 2013. "Preface." In *The Sage Handbook of Conflict Communication, Second Edition,* edited by John G. Oetzel and Stella Ting-Toomey, viii–xi. Thousand Oaks: Sage.

Panchal, Nirmita, Rabah Kamal, Cynthia Fox, and Rachel Garfield. 2021. "The Implications of COVID-19 for Mental Health and Substance Use." Accessed April 1, 2021. https://www.kff.org/coronavirus-covid-19/issue-brief/the-implications-of-covid-19-for-mental-health-and-substance-use/.

"Statement on the Second Meeting of the International Health Regulations (2005) Emergency Committee Regarding the Outbreak of Novel Coronavirus (2019-nCoV)." 2020. January 30, 2020. https://www.who.int/news/item/30-01-2020-statement-on-the-second-meeting-of-the-international-health-regulations-(2005)-emergency-committee-regarding-the-outbreak-of-novel-coronavirus-(2019-ncov).

Taylor, Derrick Bryson. "A Timeline of the Coronavirus Pandemic." *The New York Times,* March 17, 2021. https://www.nytimes.com/article/coronavirus-timeline.html.

"Who Director-General's Opening Remarks at the Media Briefing on COVID-19-11 March 2020." 2020. March 11, 2020. https://www.who.int/director-general/speeches/detail/who-director-general-s-opening-remarks-at-the-media-briefing-on-covid-19—11-march-2020.

Part I
INTIMATE COMMUNICATION

Chapter 1

Right or Wrong?

An Analysis of In-law Communication during the COVID-19 Crisis

Cara T. Mackie

Message overload and complexity ushers in fear, uncertainty, and confusion. As Coronavirus disease (COVID-19) circulated around the world in 2019–2020, anxiety followed it closely. The United States went into a safer, stay-at-home abyss for months. The U.S. Federal Government issued "slow the spread" guidelines that recommended individuals stay home for fifteen days unless absolutely necessary (White House Coronavirus Task Force "15 Days to Slow the Spread," 2020). Eventually, fifteen days turned into forty-five days (White House Coronavirus Task Force "These 30 Days," 2020). During this time, schools, stores, theme parks, beaches, movie theaters, gyms, salons, and recreation areas were closed, and restaurants closed or moved to takeout/drive-thru only. Every facet of life was in some way impacted by COVID-19. Flights, concerts, graduations, weddings, sporting events, and gatherings of ten or more people were canceled or postponed. Individuals were glued to their electronic devices, searching for confirmed case counts, death tolls, prevention tips, and the latest and up-to-date news on the virus.

The World Health Organization (WHO), Center for Disease and Prevention (CDC), and Johns Hopkins all share important information about this disease. In the beginning, these organizations shared information that sometimes reinforced each other's messages, but at times their messages conflicted. With these mixed messages, people were left wading through numbers, narratives, facts, and fictions as they tried to understand why much of the world had come to a complete halt. For some individuals, the reality of this experience centered solely around the information they consumed. Individuals clung to various interpretations of datasets, press conferences, and news stories. Media and social media have been used extensively to communicate messages about the COVID-19 pandemic (Yersel, Kalkan, and Çelen Özer 2020, 116; Zarea Gavgani 2020, 2). It became apparent that individuals re-published articles about COVID-19 on their social media accounts before evaluating the science behind the information (Zarea Gavgani 2020, 2). Due to an overabundance of information about COVID-19 shared on the internet and social media, individuals encountered an "infodemic": a rapid spread of information and misinformation (WHO "Munich Security Conference," 2020).

Not only did information and misinformation on COVID-19 flood social media outlets, information and stories about COVID-19 dominated social conversations (Reddy and Gupta 2020, 3). Berberoglu and Dinler (2021) report that exaggerated COVID-19 messages disseminated by the media were shared by friends and family, and these exchanges "played an important role in terms of generated fear" (9). These interactions with friends and family created more stress and anxiety in an already stressful time. Families are interconnected systems; therefore, stressors from this disease undoubtedly affect others in the family. Prime, Wade, and Browne (2020) suggest, maintaining one's "close relationships within the family" can help improve one's resilience during this time (638). These relationships can help individuals "weather unfavorable circumstances within the family system (or subsystems; for example, caregiver psychological distress and/or marital conflict) that may arise amid the social disruptions of COVID-19" (Prime, Wade, and Browne 2020, 638). In addition to mediated messages, one can conclude that close and personal relationships play a significant role in shaping one's perceptions about this disease.

This chapter analyzes family communication during the COVID-19 crisis, focusing on communication with in-laws. Prentice (2009) argues that it is important to study these relationships since relationships with in-laws "constitute some of the nonvoluntary relationships in which so many of us find ourselves entwined" (86). Also, in-law relationships impact other relationships within the extended family (Rittenour 2012, 94). Morr Serewicz (2014) adds, "Given that in-law relationships are often challenging, increasing understanding of these connections is a step toward easing difficulties in in-law relationships and the family more broadly" (100). Exploring the intricacies of in-law communication can lead to a better understanding of family systems.

In-law relationships form out of a marital commitment, and typically, individuals do not choose their in-laws. These relationships materialize without prior personal involvement or experiences (Rittenour 2012, 96). Thus, expectations for these relationships are formulated "based on their perceptions of others' relationships with their in-laws" (Rittenour 2012, 96), which often includes the spouse's relationship with them (Prentice 2008, 81). The family experiences a shift in family dynamics as a new member joins through marriage. Scholars suggest that a lack of schema or script for in-law communication leads to uncertainty in these relationships and an unwillingness to discuss sensitive topics (Mikucki-Enyart and Caughlin 2018, 287; Morr Serewicz 2014, 96). Mikucki-Enyart and Reed (2020) argue that there's a need in society to provide individuals with the communication tools necessary to help "manage extended family relationships" (875). Extended families are interdependent systems involving components of voluntary/involuntary and in-group/out-group dynamics.

Shantz and Hartup (1992) and Shantz and Hobart (1989) remind, "Of all interpersonal relationships, family relationships are arguably the most conflicted" (as quoted in Koerner and Fitzpatrick 2006, 164). Within family relationships, in-law relationships present distinct challenges and conflicts. Prentice (2005) states, "in-law relationships can create complex tensions in families" (6) that can be unique to in-law relationships (Prentice 2009, 72). These tensions not only affect the in-law relationship, but could impact the family system. Prentice (2009) summarizes that tensions involving loyalty, closeness, and autonomy often emerge and can problematize the relationships among in-laws (70–72). For example, a disagreement between a mother-in-law and daughter-in-law could impact the relationship between the daughter-in-law and her husband or mother and son, leaving the husband to feel as if he must choose a side. Morr Serewicz (2008) expands this notion of in-law relationships as a triad (see Duck, Foley, and Kirkpatrick 2006), reminding that the involuntary in-law relationship is often held together by the spouse or "linchpin" (265). The spouse may act as mediator between the two parties when conflict emerges. According to Morr Serewitz (2014), this triadic structure and involuntary nature of these relationships "adds layers of complexity to the interactions of in-laws" (89). During times of extreme stress, conflict may become more prevalent as families attempt to manage external stressors while negotiating the complexities of in-law communication.

Through autoethnography, the author focuses on vignettes that highlight conflict and sensemaking to better understand how families navigate(d) the COVID-19 pandemic. Ellis and Bochner (2000) describe autoethnography as introspection analyzing the interplay of self and culture/"researcher as subject" (742). Boylorn and Orbe (2020) add, autoethnography encourages "a critical lens, alongside an introspection and outward one, to make sense of who we are in the context of our cultural communities" (4). Autoethnography allows the author to critically examine interactions with in-laws through self-reflection and personal narrative. These interactions can provide insight into the impact of COVID-19 on interpersonal relationships. According to Prime, Wade, and Browne (2020), little is known about the effects COVID-19 is having on family systems and well-being (631). This research adds to the literature about family communication and in-law communication, and it further investigates the impact COVID-19 has on family systems.

IN-LAWS

May 10, 2020 (79,756 reported U.S. COVID-19 deaths, CDC)

"Where are you getting your numbers?" Sharon snarls.

"I check the World Health Organization, CDC, and Johns Hopkins websites most days," I retort.

"Well, everything I keep hearing says cases are dropping," she explains.

"Personally, I think there isn't enough testing being done so the numbers look lower, but I haven't read anything about numbers dropping," I counter.

"Oh yeah, the numbers have been going down for the last week. And there's been several stories about over reporting. A person can die in a car accident, and if she had COVID, then she is counted in the COVID deaths. In fact, instead of writing heart failure as cause of death if a person dies of heart failure while having COVID-19, they are writing coronavirus. There are monetary incentives for hospitals to write coronavirus as cause of death," she informs.

"COVID might be written on the death certificate as an underlying condition, but not the cause of death. I'm not buying it. In fact, doctors in NY are coming out against those reports, saying that would be unethical," I add.

"It is unethical," she responds.

At least, we can agree on that point. My mother-in-law and I change the subject out of respect for each other, realizing we don't agree on the severity of the COVID-19 pandemic. I try my best to let it go, but have this urge to argue. Maybe it's because I've been cooped up, maybe it's because I feel confused, or maybe it's just who I am.

August 8, 2020 (161,284 reported U.S. COVID-19 deaths, CDC)

"My mom just texted me about having dinner tonight," my partner shares.

"I don't think we will be back in time," I reply, "I thought we decided breakfast outside was the way to go? So, we aren't breathing on them in an enclosed space?"

"My parents don't care about any of that," he reminds.

"I'd feel horrible if one of us got them sick. You are still going to work and see people all the time."

"Yeah, but it's not like my mom stays home. She is still babysitting my nieces, and my sister is a nurse in a hospital. She isn't a nurse on a COVID-19 floor, but it is a large hospital in a big city. What am I going to say to my mom? We can't avoid them forever. And it's their decision to be around us. Plus, you remember what happened when we attempted breakfast outside," he adds.

"Yes, I remember," I sigh.

Our attempt to compromise: May 10, 2020. While I may have a more lackadaisical approach to my own health when it comes to COVID-19, I do try to be mindful of my seventy-plus-year-old parents and sixty-five-plus-year-old in-laws. However, they don't believe this virus is a threat to a healthy population, and they categorize themselves as a part of the healthy population. In March, when our city started to close major businesses to cut down on community spread, our college campus sent everyone home and moved to remote teaching. Without fail, as more restrictions were put into place, it seemed like my in-laws wanted to have dinner every weekend. First, we explained that it would be better to hold off on any get-togethers since I was just around hundreds of college students who had been on spring break (mostly at super spreader events). Next, we used the excuse that my husband was still going into work. Taxes are an essential business. He did have a coworker test positive. Although my husband didn't remember being in direct contact with this coworker, we still thought it wasn't worth the risk to his parents. Two weeks later, we received another invitation to dinner from his parents. "We figured if you caught it from your coworker, you would have had symptoms by now," they informed us. In an attempt to compromise, we suggested breakfast outside. It is summer in Florida so we decided on an early morning.

I thought it was a great idea. We'd eat outside and enjoy nature, plus get to visit. And keep a safe distance. We brought our own outdoor chairs, coffee, and silverware. While we waited for his dad to arrive with food, we set up a place for us to eat. They'd been ordering breakfast from a local diner to support local businesses every weekend. We agree with the idea of supporting local businesses, but we had not been eating out while in the midst of a pandemic. Maybe we were being too cautious. We agreed on takeout for breakfast.

Scene

The morning air still has some coolness to it. The birds are just waking up, and we watch a Cardinal flickering in an oak tree. We talk with my mother-in-law, trying to avoid politics or COVID-19. My father-in-law arrives, and we wave at him as he brings the food into the house. My mother-in-law heads indoors to grab the food and napkins. She walks out with her long sleeves covering her hands as she balances the containers with our meals. We rush to help her.

"I was going to wear gloves, but I figured I could cover my hands with my sleeves. Since, I know you don't want me touching your meals," she states.

I glance at my husband. She walks back in to get her meal.

"What is she talking about? Does she realize that all of our caution is for them, not us?"

My husband shrugs.

My mother-in-law returns with her meal. And we begin to eat. Of course, we can't ignore the state of affairs, and her and I begin to argue about research on COVID-19 and treatment. My husband chimes in, "How was your trip to the park with Stephanie (his niece)?" He manages to shift the tension in the air, and we talk about family. As the sun begins to creep over the oak tree, we finish breakfast and wrap-up our visit. My father-in-law did not join us. He didn't even come out to say, "hi."

"What just happened?" I ask as we drive away, "Your dad could have at least said 'it's too hot outside for me to join you but good to see you both.' I am in awe that he didn't acknowledge our visit."

My husband doesn't say much. It seems as if he wants to laugh at me. He grew up with his dad, and he knows him well. My mother-in-law is a retired nurse and my father-in-law is a retired medical doctor. This puts them in a unique position to interpret the information about COVID-19 from a medical lens. They think this virus only threatens those who fall into vulnerable population.

September 13, 2020 (193,705 reported U.S. COVID-19 deaths, CDC)

As we plate our buffet-style dinner, my mother-in-law asks us several questions about our summer road trip from Lakeland, FL to Denver, CO. My family met in Denver to visit my brother. Once out in CO, we spent much of our visit hiking various CO trails. I explain to my in-laws that one of the hiking trails required us to our wear face masks when passing others. My mom was with us on this hike, and she was having a hard time breathing through her mask. We were hiking vertical climbs at a higher altitude, and at seventy-one, mom was getting out of breath. Her mask made her feel claustrophobic, and she was on the verge of a panic attack. She decided against donning the mask during the rest of the hike. We stopped along the way to let her catch her breath and decided we would move to the edge of the trail when individuals passed us. Since my mom was having a hard time breathing, she would face away from any passerby (instead of putting on a mask). However, one lady said a very rude comment about my mom's lack of a mask. *You don't know anything about our situation*, I thought. My mother replied, "It's such a beautiful day out." As I finish this story, my mother-in-law shares her thoughts on mask mandates.

"I have a letter from my doctor stating that I am medically exempt from wearing a mask due to health issues. It is an ADA violation to ask for more information about my health. If a person has a problem with me, then I show the letter. The truth is that masks can be detrimental and don't allow for adequate oxygen," she explains.

"I have a very difficult time with masks. Since I have asthma, I already have a hard-enough time breathing. When I wear a mask I sometimes feel panic. But I am trying to teach for an hour and forty minutes in a mask. It is a long time. I've tried many types and styles of masks but nothing changes the fact that I can't breathe," I reply.

"I refuse to wear one," she says, "there are many contradictory research articles out there on efficacy."

"In fact, research on flu viruses and masks report masks provide no protection for either party," my father-in-law interjects.

"I think staying far away from a person is the best bet," I attempt a half-joke.

"The mask mandates are a way to test out how much of the population can be manipulated and controlled. This gives them a good gage to see if they can control people. I refuse to be a sheep. I will not give into a mandate that has no scientific backing to it. When I see all these people in masks, it is so upsetting. I think don't be a sheep. Don't be a follower," she begins.

"I'm not sure how I feel about masks, yet. I would think that if a person who has the virus sneezes or coughs, then some of the spray would be caught in the mask. But I don't think masks are going to entirely stop the spread of COVID as some would have you believe," I add.

"No, they are worse. Because people constantly touch and adjust their masks, and then they touch their eyes. Masks could create more problems, and most people don't wear a mask that would stop anything from spreading," my father-in-law responds.

"I do wear a mask sometimes, like in a check-out line where I am closer to others, out of respect to those around me. I would hate to be spreading the virus without knowing it," I say.

"I don't. If I am not feeling well, then I don't go out. Everyone needs to wash their hands. And often times asymptomatic people aren't the ones spreading the virus. In fact, if a person looks at me funny for not wearing a mask or has something to say, then they are asking for me to cough on them," she coughs and leans over, acting this out.

I laugh in an uncomfortable way, and my partner and I look at each other. He remains quiet during this entire conversation. I realize that his silence is my cue to stop encouraging this topic of conversation. And my partner attempts to change the conversation. I am shocked to see my mother-in-law reenact coughing on someone. It seems extreme. I am reminded how odd it is that mask shaming is common nowadays. I've heard mask shaming occur when a group of people who don't wear a mask because they disagree with a mask mandate make those who wear a mask feel judged. And it can occur when a group of people who do wear masks because they believe in a mask mandate make those who don't wear a mask feel judged. A small piece of material can create such divide.

January 29, 2021 (435,151 reported U.S. COVID-19 deaths, CDC)

I listen. And silently disagree. I listen. And become afraid that the opinion being shared by my colleague would be accepted as the opinion of all faculty. I listen. I want to say, *but this will not be mandatory, right?* I listen:

"Is the college doing anything to get faculty recognized as 'teachers' in order to get us on the list for the first round of vaccines?" my colleague inquires, "I mean, we are on the front lines, in the classroom, potentially being exposed to the vaccine."

Are we on the "front lines"? In most classrooms, we are at teaching stations situated in the front of the class quite far from the students. I listen:

"Florida seems very behind in the vaccine rollout. I know the government is trying to get everyone 65+ vaccinated first, but in Florida that is a very tall order. They don't have enough vaccines for that let alone for others," she continues.

"I know in Polk Country they are starting to vaccinate public school teachers," another faculty member adds.

"We are trying to work with the local hospitals, clinics, and really anyone who will listen to get the college employees recognized as a population who should get the vaccine now," an administrator replies, "But so far no luck. The most promising outcome we've heard includes getting nursing students who are participating in their clinicals vaccinated. Although, we haven't seen this happen, yet."

Are we really spending fifteen minutes talking about the vaccine? This topic has nothing to do with our meeting or the agenda. I listen:

"Once the vaccine is more widely available, are there going to be policies in place for students or individuals working at the college?" the first faculty asks.

"So far, this has not been discussed," the administrator affirms.

Should I speak up? Should I say something—not everyone is comfortable with the vaccine. I scan the Zoom call participants. I can't be the only one on this call that is hesitant about the vaccine. A vaccine we have no long-term data to review.

I listen to three out of the eight faculty in this meeting engage in a conversation about the importance of receiving this vaccine. I don't know why I don't speak up just to clarify that not all faculty would get the vaccine if offered. I don't want to get into a debate. I respect one's decision to be vaccinated. Maybe, I am in the silent majority. But in this setting surrounded by colleagues, I don't want to be the outcast. I feel my credibility as an intellectual capable of reading and understanding scientific research would be smashed.

I am worried I'd be judged. *I am tired of justifying and quoting all the research that I have been reading. I often wonder if the individuals who I frequently disagree with are reading research or parroting "fact-check" websites.*

When I finish this meeting, I share my concerns with my partner. To this he responds:

"Well, my mom just called me to warn me about the vaccine. She was extremely serious and wanted to make sure we weren't going to get it. She said to call my dad, if we have any questions. Apparently, there are studies that are not being discussed by the media that my dad has been reading. These articles detail out the side-effects (which include death) and the ineffectiveness of the vaccine."

"Wait, why would your mom call you to convince you to not get it? We never said we would get it," I ask, "doesn't she trust us to make our own informed decision?"

"Nope, something must have gotten her worked up about it," he adds.

"I'm not an anti-vaxxer, but I believe in doing one's homework and making educated decisions about which vaccines to get. I'm still trying to interpret the research on this vaccine," I reflect.

"It's my mom and dad," he concludes.

"They already expressed their opinions about the vaccine to us two other times. In fact, I think each time we've seen them since the release of the vaccine they've shared their opinions with us," I remind.

"I know. And I am sure the next time we see them, they will repeat it," he nods.

"At least your mom and I stopped arguing about the severity of the disease, and they stopped teaching us about the harmful effects of masks. But now we have to hear about vaccines. At some point, all this makes it harder to want to visit with them," I add.

"I do think we have to be careful about family gatherings again. Since the COVID numbers have spiked, hospitals are getting overloaded. And little is known about the newer variants of this virus. I hope they can respect our decision to avoid gathering right now," he concludes.

"Maybe. Probably not."

Moving forward, I doubt I will share my opinions on the virus with my in-laws. *I am tired of justifying and quoting all the research that I have been reading. I often wonder if the individuals who I frequently disagree with are reading research or parroting "conspiracies theory" websites.*

TRAVERSING CONFLICT

Dialectical Tensions

As my in-laws and I navigated conversations on COVID-19, we began to renegotiate dialectical tensions of autonomy-connection, predictability-novelty, and openness-closedness (Baxter 1990; Baxter and Montgomery 1996, 4–5). I wanted to spend time with my in-laws, but the overwhelming disagreements we had about the virus created a desire for independence. There were times when I would have to mentally prepare myself before a visit with my in-laws, knowing we would end up discussing COVID-19. COVID-19 brought new attention to these competing desires and has shifted the discussion on the autonomy-connection dialectic from competing desires to needs. Frequently, my desire for autonomy became a need for separation out of worry or concern for my in-laws. My in-laws are in their late sixties, and while considered healthy, they belong to a vulnerable population. Many times, my partner explained to his parents that we would hate to get them sick. We were not avoiding them, but out of caution wanted to maintain distance. It seemed as if my mother-in-law internalized our approach to the virus as offensive. She interpreted our caution to visit them as we did not want to see them. We viewed it as we were protecting them. Eventually, their desire for closeness outweighed our need for independence.

Part of my mother-in-law's desire for connection stemmed from the predictably of our visits pre-COVID-19. Our desires for predictability and novelty include an uneasiness with uncertainty (Baxter and Montgomery 1996, 5). COVID-19 has upheaved our notions of certainty and spontaneity, creating uncertainty on many levels. Prior to COVID-19, dinner with my in-laws was a predictable event. We did not have set dates for dinner, and we could be somewhat spontaneous. But the act of dinner was predictable. Since we live less than five miles from my in-laws, every few weeks we would have dinner with them (pre-COVID-19). My need for independence disrupted the predictability of our dinner plans. This disruption created unease. My mother-in-law repeatedly asked us over for dinner in an attempt to restore predictability. The act of saying no created even more tension. This led to an influx of pressure from my in-laws for us to see the virus as a non-threat.

My partner's email was inundated with email attachments on research and commentary about the virus from his father. Each article supported his parents' stance on the virus. As the pandemic stretched from weeks to months, my desire to avoid conflict with my in-laws impacted how often I shared my perspective on the virus. According to Mikucki-Enyart and Caughlin (2018), "children-in-law may prefer to avoid potentially precarious discussions" to help cope with relational uncertainty (286). In the beginning, I had many open conversations about COVID-19 with my mother-in-law, but it became apparent early on that we may not always agree with each other. We began to negotiate the openness-closedness dialectic. *How much do I share with my in-laws?* As a daughter-in-law, I found this difficult to navigate. I did not want to create problems in my marriage or with my in-laws. I have known my in-laws for almost ten years, but I am still learning how to adjust to their family.

Their family communication style is drastically different than mine. My family is almost too open, and my partner's family is almost too closed. After one of our first disagreements about COVID-19, my mother-in-law apologized for being combatant. I explained that I did not view it as combatant and appreciated a good debate. I also apologized, knowing I can be very argumentative. Through this experience, I learned that a "lack of openness is as necessary as openness to the wellbeing" of our relationship (Baxter and Montgomery 1996, 5). I started to just listen to my in-laws discuss the virus, but kept most of my views to myself. I constantly renegotiated a "need not to talk and need to talk" (Baxter and Montgomery 1996, 6). My desires for closedness and openness forced me to reflect on my communication style and conflict management skills.

Managing Tensions

My in-laws are medical professionals, and I am not. One dilemma I encountered when processing the tensions with my in-laws involved my internal conflict to question their perceptions on the virus. My in-laws are more qualified in this area than I. *Who am I to challenge them?* I did not always disagree with them on every point about the virus. In fact, I often agreed with them. However, these moments of disagreement seemed to have more power. These moments defined and refined my relationship with my in-laws. *How do you argue with a medical doctor when you are just a consumer of information? You don't. You just listen.* During many conversations with my in-laws, I retreated into silence in attempt to satisfy my need for closedness. And this silence allowed me to be present. I began to truly listen to them. Not necessarily agree, but listen.

I learned that mindful listening was the most effective communication skill I used while negotiating the above tensions. Shafir (2006) writes, "Mindful listening allows us to do more than take in people's words; it helps us better understand the how and why of their views" (12). The more I practiced mindful listening, the more I learned about my in-laws. My mother-in-law continued to "plan" (Prentice, Zeidan, and Wang 2020, 4) and maintain her norm to better adjust to the stressors associate with COVID-19. I began to see my in-laws' persistence on predictability, connection, and openness as a way of coping with the uncertainty of the virus.

Mindful listening is a way to "manage emotional vulnerability" between parties (Ting-Toomey and Dorjee 2019, 229). This pandemic has created emotional vulnerability for all of us on many levels. As I better understood their perspective, I felt less inclined to engage in conflict with them. Shafir (2006) continues, "When understanding occurs, a sense of calm is achieved on both sides, even if no point of agreement is reached" (12). Since my in-laws are medical professionals, I believe that when I did disagree with them about COVID-19 it was more personal. I was not just inciting a debate, but insulting their training in medicine (which I was not). Frequently, my mother-in-law would remind me that my father-in-law is a medical doctor and has found several research articles about the virus that he would like me to read. By listening mindfully, I began to validate their thoughts and feelings and restore trust in them as professionals. I was reminded that "from understanding, respect and trust for one another are possible" (Shafir 2006, 12).

REFLECTIONS

In the beginning of the COVID-19 debates, I was genuinely confused about the "us vs. them" attitude. *How many arguments about COVID-19 did I engage? How many times did I have to say in an argument that I read an interesting article about the flu and wearing a mask (Cowling et al. 2010) which helped me formulate my opinion on masks?* I remember calling my dad to talk more about this (mis)information overload. We spoke about research on COVID-19, mask mandates, and politics. We analyzed various contentions that emerged between friends and family due to COVID-19. During this conversation, my dad shared that unfortunately politics and one's own agenda will cloud truth and fact. And everyone has "proof" on their side. I feel like the public information we receive about COVID-19 is a patchwork of guesses.

This "infodemic" forced me to dig and dig for peer-reviewed scientific articles. I still feel quite confused by the quick turnaround on these peer-reviewed journal articles. *Shouldn't these studies take longer to conduct and longer to review?* I've immersed myself in so much data but surfaced feeling misinformed. Redden (2020) states, COVID-19 research articles are getting pushed to the top of review piles, hence the quick turnaround. However, she points to open-access "preprint" studies (studies uploaded before a peer-reviewed process is completed) as a factor in the quick release of information. Redden (2020) cautions this practice, noting the flaws in some of the research and the retractions of COVID-19 articles in progress. As more (mis) information emerged, I found myself discussing it with colleagues, friends, and family.

I noticed a difference between the conversations about COVID-19 with my family and the conversations about COVID-19 with my in-laws. When talking with my in-laws about COVID-19, there was an intensity about it. And it could get preachy: they are right and that is that. When I disagreed with my in-laws, I felt judged by them (as in the May 10th conversation above). They tried their hardest to get me to change my mind about the virus. Prentice (2009) finds that an "expressing approval/withholding judgement" dialectic emerged during initial stages of in-laws communication (80). She states, "Thus parents were caught in a dialectical tension of how much approval of the potential spouse to communicate before engagement or marriage" (81). I found that this tension could reemerge throughout various stages of in-law relationships, especially during stressful life events. As in-laws decide whether or not they approve or disapprove of the couple's situation or life choices, they become uncertain about how to relate to their daughter/son-in-law. We may find ourselves renegotiating "family in-group" status (Morr Serewicz 2014, 99). I felt like my parents listened to my thoughts about COVID-19, and there was a sense of your interpretation and mine. Both could be right, but both could be wrong.

I realize that my strong identification with my family could impact my ability to identify with my in-laws. According to Rittenour and Soliz (2009), "Expectations of specific communication behaviors" could be "associated with family-of-origin" and create potential communication barriers (86). When discussing COVID-19, my parents listened to me. They did not always agree with me, but I never felt as if they passed judgment. At times, I forget that my family communication pattern with my immediate family influences my expectations for my in-law communication ("high conversation orientation" vs. "low conversation orientation"). I have to reevaluate these expectations and remember my in-laws and I have a different communication style. I'm learning to adjust my communication style to better fit each interaction.

Navigating a relationship with my in-laws during COVID-19 required me to negotiate dialectical tensions, practice conflict management, and reevaluate my communication style. Prentice (2005) states, "relational dialectics can add insights into the process that people go through as they [re]produce the structures and routines of their family lives" (34). Managing these tensions through listening allowed me to better understand my partner's family and communication patterns. In turn, this experience created opportunities for my partner and I to have an open dialogue about our families' influence on our individual communication styles. My partner and I do not always agree with each other when discussing COVID-19, but we do respect each other. We do agree that COVID-19 has created a strain on our relationship with his parents. As COVID-19 lingers, most people are starting to feel COVID-19 burn-out. Unfortunately, this disease will be around for a while. Fortunately, mindful listening is a communication tool that shows investment in the relationship and creates a shared understanding. This pandemic highlights the importance of effective communication in all areas of our life, especially interpersonally.

REFERENCES

Baxter, Leslie A. 1990. "Dialectical Contradictions in Relationship Development." *Journal of Social and Personal Relationships* 7 (1) (February): 69–88. https://doi.org/10.1177/0265407590071004.

Baxter, Leslie A. and Barbara M. Montgomery.1996. *Relating: Dialogues and Dialectics*. United Kingdom: Guilford Publications.

Berberoglu, Aysen and Asim Dinler. 2021. "The Mediator Role of Communication about COVID-19 on the Relationship between Exaggeration of Media and Generated Fear: Case of North Cyprus." *Journal of Clinical and Experimental Investigations* 12 (1): 1–9, article em00759. https://doi.org/10.29333/jcei/9281.

Boylorn, Robin M. and Mark P. Orbe. 2020. "Introduction: Critical Autoethnography as Method of Choice." In *Critical Autoethnography*, second edition, edited by Robin Boylorn and Mark Orbe, 1–18. New York, NY: Routledge.

CDC, n.d. "Trends in Number of COVID-19 Cases and Deaths in the US Reported to CDC, by State/Territory." Accessed January 30, 2021. https://covid.cdc.gov/covid-data-tracker/#trends_totalandratedeaths.

Cowling, B. J., Y. Zhou, D. K. M. Ip, G. M. Leung, and A. E. Aiello. 2010. "Face Masks to Prevent Transmission of Influenza Virus: A Systematic Review." *Epidemiology and Infection* 138 (4): 449–56. https://doi.org/10.1017/S0950268809991658.

Duck, Steven, Megan K. Foley, and D. Charles Kirkpatrick. 2006. "Relating Difficulty in a Triangular World." In *Relating Difficulty: The Processes of Constructing and Managing Difficult Interaction*, edited by D. Charles Kirkpatrick, Steven Duck, and Megan K. Foley, 225–32. Mahwah, NJ: Lawrence Erlbaum Associates.

Ellis, Carolyn and Arthur Bochner. 2000. Autoethnography, Personal Narrative, Reflectivity: Researcher as Subject." In *Handbook of Qualitative Research*, second edition, edited by Norman Denzin and Yvonna Lincoln, 733–68. Thousand Oaks, CA: Sage Publishing.

Johns Hopkins University & Medicine, n.d. "Tracking." Accessed November 20, 2020. https://coronavirus.jhu.edu/data.

Koerner, Ascan F. and Mary Anne Fitzpatrick. 2006. "Family Conflict Communication." In *The Sage Handbook of Conflict Communication,* edited by John Oetzel and Stella Ting-Toomey, 159–83. http://dx.doi.org/10.4135/9781412976176.n6.

Mikucki-Enyart, Sylvia L. and Jaclyn M. Reed. 2020. "Understanding Parents-in-Law's Uncertainty Management through a Relational Turbulence Lens." *Communication Studies* 71 (5): 857–78. https://doi.org/10.1080/10510974.2020.1776745.

Mikucki-Enyart, Sylvia L. and John P. Caughlin. 2018. "Integrating the Relational Turbulence Model and a Multiple Goals Approach to Understand Topic Avoidance during Transition to Extended Family." *Communication Research* 45 (3): 267–96. https://doi.org/10.1177%2F0093650215595075.

Morr Serewicz, Mary Claire. 2008. "Toward a Triangular Theory of the Communication and Relationships of In-Laws: Theoretical Proposal and Social Relations Analysis of Relational Satisfaction and Private Disclosure in In-Law Triads." *Journal of Family Communication* 8: 264–92. https://doi.org/10.1080/15267430802397161.

———. 2014. "Relationship With Parents-in-law." In *Widening the Family Circle: New Research on Family Communication,* second edition, edited by Kory Floyd and Mark T. Morman, 85–101. Thousand Oaks, CA: Sage Publications.

Prentice, Carolyn M. 2005. "The Assimilation of In-laws: The Impact of Newcomers on the Structuration of Families." PhD diss., University of Missouri-Columbia.

———. 2008. "The Assimilation of In-Laws: The Impact of Newcomers on the Communication Routines of Families." *Journal of Applied Communication Research* 36 (1): 74–97. https://doi.org/10.1080/00909880701799311.

———. 2009. "Relational Dialectics Among In-Laws." *Journal of Family Communication* 9 (2) (April–June): 67–89. https://doi.org/10.1080/15267430802561667.

Prentice, Catherine, Susan Zeidan, and Xuequn Wang. 2020. "Personality, Trait EI and Coping with COVID 19 Measures." *International Journal of Disaster Risk Reduction* 51 (December): 1–10, article 101789. https://doi.org/10.1016/j.ijdrr.2020.101789.

Prime, Heather, Mark Wade, and Dillion Browne. 2020. "Risk and Resilience in Family Well-Being during the COVID-19 Pandemic." *American Psychologist* 75 (5), 631–643. https://doi.org/10.1037/amp0000660.

Redden, Elizabeth. 2020. "Rush to Publish Risks Undermining COVID-19 Research." *Inside Higher Ed,* June 8, 2020. https://www.insidehighered.com/news/2020/06/08/fast-pace-scientific-publishing-covid-comes-problems.

Reddy, B. Venkatashiva and Arti Gupta. 2020. "Importance of Effective Communication during COVID-19 Infodemic." *Journal of Family Medicine & Primary Care* 9 (8) (August): 3793–3796.

Rittenour, Christine. 2012. "Daughter-in-law Standards for Mother-in-law Communication: Associations With Daughter-in-law Perceptions of Relational Satisfaction and Shared Family Identity." *Journal of Family Communication* 12: 93–110. https://doi.org/10.1080/15267431.2010.537240.

Rittenour, Christine and Jordan Soliz. 2009. "Communicative and Relational Dimensions of Shared Family Identity and Relational Intentions in Mother-in-Law/Daughter-in-Law Relationships: Developing a Conceptual Model for Mother-in-Law/Daughter-in-Law Research." *Western Journal of Communication* 73 (1): 67–90. https://doi.org/10.1080/10570310802636334.

Shafir, Rebecca Z. 2006. *Communication in the Age of Distraction.* Wheaton, IL: Quest Books.

Ting-Toomey, Stella and Tenzin Dorjee. 2019. *Communicating Across Cultures*, second edition. New York, NY: The Guilford Press.

White House Coronavirus Task Force. March 16, 2020. "15 Days to Slow the Spread." Accessed February 27, 2021. https://trumpwhitehouse.archives.gov/articles/15-days-slow-spread/.

———. April 2, 2020. "These 30 Days: How You Can Help." Accessed February 27, 2021. https://trumpwhitehouse.archives.gov/articles/these-30-days-how-you-can-help/.

World Health Organization. n.d. "Coronavirus Disease (COVID-19) Pandemic." Accessed November 20, 2020. https://covid19.who.int.

———. February, 15 2020. "Munich Security Conference." Accessed February 10, 2021. https://www.who.int/director-general/speeches/detail/munich-security-conference.

Yersel, Burcin, Başak Kalkan, and Arzu Çelen Özer. 2020. "An Evaluation on Social Media Content Strategies of Expert Opinion Leaders Working in the Healthcare Field during the COVID-19 Pandemic Process." *Usak University Journal of Social Sciences* 2: 115–29. https://dergipark.org.tr/tr/pub/usaksosbil/issue/59466/814335.

Zarea Gavgani, Vahideh. 2020. "Infodemic in the Global Coronavirus Crisis." *Depiction of Health* 11 (1): 1–5. http://dohweb.tbzmed.ac.ir.

Chapter 2

Talking Myself off a Ledge

Navigating Identity during COVID-19 Quarantine

Pamela Dykes

How does one remain calm when the words *crisis, isolation, pandemic, quarantine, fear,* and *death* are fed to us on a daily basis? It has been hard to remain calm during the COVID-19 pandemic. COVID-19 has exacerbated mental health problems, such as anxiety and depression, and created a global economic recession (Buttell, et al. 2021,1). Many people are feeling the impact of COVID-related stress and depression. In addition to experiencing emotional tensions, there were other collective challenges faced by individuals during the pandemic (Stamps, 2021, 134). For example, Black people, in particular were confronted with what the author perceived as "global anti-Blackness."

In this chapter, the author explores ideological shifts experienced during quarantine. The goal of this research is to explore the author's personal narratives and the communicative themes that emerged. Through the self-reflective process of autoethnography, the researcher investigates the narrative experiences of a mother and caregiver during the early months of the COVID-19 Crisis. This study reveals how the author's identity fluctuated while being sandwiched between young adult children and an elderly parent during quarantine. The author also reported feeling a heightened sense of connectedness to her racial identity during this time.

RESEARCH APPROACH AND THEORY

Autoethnography

Autoethnography is the research approach used to analyze this piece, because of its reflexive nature, where the researcher is inserted into the research. This method was used to help the author make sense of cultural and personal experiences. Ellis, Adams, and Bochner (2015) explain, "autoethnography combines characteristic of *auto*biography and *ethno*graphy" (2). Additionally, they describe autoethnography as "autobiographies that self-consciously explore the interplay of the introspective, personally engaged self with cultural descriptions mediated through language" (742). This method allows the researcher to insert autobiographical accounts of critical moments in one's life while gathering research. This grasp of the self is essential when considering the researcher's position adapted while analyzing others. This enables (me) the researcher to discuss preconceived beliefs and biases while on the research journey. Using this method also "values relationships with others" (1), which was an integral aspect of this study.

To understand experiences in quarantine, the author conducted a narrative analysis of journal entries collected between the months of March 2020 through July 2020, which revealed two themes. The first theme looks at how the author grappled with perceived "super woman expectations" of family members, and the second theme focuses on personal struggles, including racial identity. In addition to using an autoethnographic narrative analysis, the theoretical frame employed for this study is the Communication Theory of Identity. My idea "of self (who am I)" was in a constant state of flux.

COMMUNICATION THEORY OF IDENTITY

Derived from Social Identity Theory, the Communication Theory of Identity (CTI) posits that identity emerges as a result of social interaction, ascription, and interpersonal construction of one's experiences (Hecht, et al. 2003). CTI also asserts that identity is a naturally communicative and relational phenomenon (Hecht et al. 2005, 259). Communication builds, sustains, and transforms identity. At the same time, identity is expressed through communication (259). The CTI posits four layers of identity (personal, enacted, relational, and communal) that can be observed through qualitative research (Upshaw, 2021, 4). CTI has been studied from multiple perspectives. For example, Upshaw (2021) utilized CTI to explicate salient identities among African American prostate cancer survivors (5), while Rubinski (2019) used CTI to research jealousy in polyamorous relationships (17). Rubinski (2019) found that identity occurs through interaction with others and that jealousy is an identity-laden relational situation in polyamorous relationships (18). In another study, Wagner (2017) used CTI to find the misalignment between the personal, relational, and enacted frames in men who pursue extreme fitness goals (1), and identified three identity gaps: excessive body discipline, forceful negotiation, and constant comparison (1).

It is clear that CTI has been studied in many different realms; however, it has not been specifically used to frame COVID-19 experiences. Thus, the goal of this study is to add to the identity literature by using CTI to guide a narrative analysis of journal entries that highlight personal identity shifts experienced by the author during quarantine. To get a better understanding of this phenomenon a sampling of the journal entries is provided below.

JOURNAL ENTRIES

Journal Entry One: February Early Rumblings

I walk into the communication building at Florida Southern College past the large TV mounted on the wall, and I can hear the CNN news anchors talking about some sickness in China. They were talking about it being some type of flu that was highly contagious and right now there was no cure for it. While I stood there my co-worker walked up to me and says, "I have a feeling this is going to be bad!"

"Nah, it's going to be exactly like all of the other viruses that were sensationalized in the past. The Bird Flu, the West Nile Virus, Ebola, the Zika Virus and the Swine Flu which two of my children actually contracted. They had a high fever for two or three days accompanied by vomiting, but it was over in about a week," I reply.

"I don't know, Pam. I think it is going to be much worse," she explains.

"This virus is going to be exactly like those outbreaks where the media makes a huge deal about it and then 'poof' it's gone. We don't hear any more about the virus or sickness that was threatening humanity," I say. We continue to glare at the news report.

"No! This is going to be different. My husband and I are bracing for the impact of this. We have ordered as many masks as we can because they are becoming scarce, and the price has gone up on them over the past couple of months. This virus is deadly, and it is killing lots of people abroad," she lectures.

The key word here is "abroad." There are only a few cases in the United States. The President swears we only have fifteen cases, and those fifteen cases are going to go away. Shouldn't I believe him? We should be safe? Right?

Journal Entry Two: Class is in Session for EVERYONE

I woke up on Tuesday morning to multiple voices. I think they are coming from my son Brysen's room. I take a shower, get dressed, and go to his room to see who was in my home. When I open the door to Brysen's room I hear "Mom!" from four young men. Only one of them was my child. Brysen's three best friends were over because the WIFI was "acting up at the crib," so Zach had to come to my house to complete his college coursework. I also hear more screaming/yelling so I close that door and go to my son, Braelen's room. His room was my old office that I converted into a bedroom when my father moved in with me last summer. I go to his room, and he is sitting on the edge of his bed, shirtless in his signature basketball shorts, playing a video game. He is not aware that he is yelling because he has headphones on and doesn't know how loud he sounds. However, it sounds like he is yelling to me. I tell him to quiet down, and I ask him when he has to attend class. He says at 12:00 p.m. I close the door and check in on my daughter Belicia. I open her door to find her sitting on her bed in the dark (because she still has her Black out drapes closed), listening to her instructor lecture on Zoom. *CRAP! How am I going to conduct my classes with all of this noise and all of these people in my home?* I am also concerned because it doesn't seem like my son is taking this seriously. Technically, we are not allowed to have people who are outside of our family in our home. Young people never take things seriously. I close the refrigerator door where I was standing, drinking my cold brew coffee from the bottle, contemplating where I am going to teach my classes. Then I go to my room and stage my make shift classroom because it is the only quiet place in my home.

Journal Entry Three: The Walls Are Caving In

It has been more than a month since we have been sheltering at home, and I feel like I am going stir crazy. Years ago, I can remember watching a news program that reported on the idea that many people, especially baby boomers, were part of the sandwich generation, which is the idea that people will still be raising children while caring for aging parents. I knew this could end up being me because I delayed having children until my thirties, and my paternal grandparents lived to be 102. I also knew that our family as a whole tries to take care of our elderly unless it is medically impossible to do so. Although my brothers and I had arranged for my parents to live with my younger brother, my dad moved in with me one year ago due to unforeseen events. Although we had discussed a different plan, I always knew my dad would end up with me in the end.

I spend most days in my bedroom in between trips downstairs to cook and do the cleaning for my family. Although I live with four other people, I am beginning to feel lonelier than I have ever felt before. Although I have a house full of people, I think the loneliness comes from the feeling that I am the only adult in the house, even though there are another three people in the home who are considered adults. My sons who are twenty-one and nineteen and my dad who is eighty-two are all adults in the traditional sense. Even though they are all grown, everyone in the home looks at me as the protector, decision-maker, provider, and yes mother, even to my dad. This is beginning to feel like a heavyweight. I am beginning to get weary and exhausted.

This feeling of loneliness is exacerbated while watching my sons entertaining their girlfriends in our family room. I watch them cook pizza, make brownies, and drink wine in our nice wine glasses. I laughed to myself. *Are they on a date in my living room and didn't offer me anything? That's rude.* I raised my kids to understand that it was rude to eat in front of people without offering it to them. I would have said no but they should have asked. I talk myself off the ledge reminding myself I would have done the same thing at that age. You don't really know how to be a caretaker until you become a parent. They don't know any better but they will understand once they have families of their own. My dad, on the other hand, is completely different than us, and I have to remember that he grew up in a completely different time. Men worked outside of the home, and women worked inside the home doing all of the housework: the cooking and cleaning. I have to remember that my mom waited on him hand and foot. However, I know he at least knows how to make a peanut butter sandwich on toast and fix his favorite cereal. Although my dad grew up in a different time, I couldn't understand why he didn't learn how to cook anything. His brothers knew how to cook, and I remember my grandfather cooking breakfast, vegetable soup, fried potatoes, peach cobbler. We enjoyed my grandfather's famous eggnog every Christmas. Oh well, my dad was such a good father to me while I was growing up, and I promised my mother I would take good care of him.

Journal Entry Four: Cabin Fever and Quarantine Fatigue

While lying in my bed at night, I can't stop thinking about how mothered I feel while living in this house with the weight of the world sitting on my chest. I feel the impact psychologically, emotionally, and physically because of my asthma. On one hand, I desperately want to leave the house and do all of the things I used to do. However, with my underlying conditions, I know that it would be wise to stay at home. On a daily basis I find myself trying to manage how to keep our home clean and sterile in order to keep my father safe. I could not imagine my father in a hospital alone gasping for air on a ventilator. Then on May 25, 2020, I watch George Floyd die on television pleading for his life stating, "I can't breathe." *This is so sad.* We are going from bad to worse. We have been fighting an invisible respiratory virus, and now we are fighting another type of virus, but this one attacks the heart of humanity. In that very moment I shift from: I can't wait until I get outside where I can freely smile and breathe without the confinement of my mask, to now I'm afraid to leave the house because my family members are more likely to die of COVID-19, or at the hands of a rogue police officer than my white counterparts. *What in the world is going on?* I am afraid, battling cabin fever, and I'm beginning to feel depressed.

Journal Entry Five: Is COVID-19 Over?

It's been almost three weeks since George Floyd died, and I haven't heard anything about the virus. In one day, we went from having endless media updates about infected COVID-19 cases and deaths to continuous news about racial tensions. In the past couple of weeks there have been constant videos of racial protests held all over the county and the world, including the unfortunate pictures of looting and the burning down of police stations near the site of Floyd's death. Also, news outlets have continued to replay the horrific video showing the police officers arresting George and then later killing him by asphyxiation. George was held down, handcuffed on the ground with two police officers putting their body weight on him. One of them held him down with his knee on his neck for almost nine minutes while several bystanders cried for his release. Some bystanders videotaped this part of his arrest. I am feeling really depressed and very scared. As an African American woman and a mother, all I can think about is that could have been one of my sons, nephews, brothers, father, and/or friends.

My heart is broken, and I am very weary. The sad thing is that this incident was not an isolated event. There are many cases that have been recorded over the past couple of years. I believe that these brutal killings have been going on from slavery to present day. The difference between now and then is the fact that people have caught this violence on video. I felt like we were actually experiencing two crises in this country: one around the COVID-19 pandemic and the other around the racial divide and the systematic oppression of people of color. One afternoon, I was talking with someone about these current events, and this person said that racial inequity has nothing to do with the COVID-19 pandemic. I think it does because it has been rumored that people of color account for the majority of cases. For example, according to reports, George Floyd actually tested positive for COVID-19 before his death (Karimi and Fox 2020, 1). It is all so saddening and sickening. As I watch one of the videos on TV, I notice that most of those people have masks on and now all of the protests appear to be peaceful. I feel very torn when I see the protests on TV. I feel like I should be there but I'm afraid I don't want to infect anyone, and

I don't want to contract this virus either. This is such a crazy time—a CRAP SHOW if you ask me but I know that we will all get through it somehow.

Journal Entry Six: COVID-19 Back in The News

June tenth is the day after George Floyd's funeral and memorial services. The news media is back to reporting information about COVID-19. It's very interesting and scary. We have started to reopen in Florida. The governor is calling it Phase One which means restaurants are allowed to open with the recommended CDC guidelines (mask and social distancing). I really don't feel comfortable leaving the house because I don't think Florida really fits the criteria to begin opening things up. There still isn't a vaccine, and we still know very little about the virus. The information about the virus changes every day. *How will I keep everyone in my house safe when the government is telling us to go out and spend money? I know some people will die but somebody's got to take the hit, hopefully, it won't be you or anyone you know.* Okay, that is not what the officials actually are saying but that is the sentiment or the way I feel about it.

DISCUSSION

I identify with the notion of "identity gaps," and aimed to explore this idea through narrative analysis. During quarantine, I journaled between the months of March 2020 and July 2020. At the end of each day, I recorded what was going on in the world and how it was impacting me. I touched upon many subjects such as fear, isolation, anger, and what it was like to be sheltering in place with my family. This narrative analysis revealed identity fluctuations I experienced while in quarantine with an elderly parent and my three young adult children. Two identity themes emerged from the analysis: (1) the impact of caregiving on the author's identity as the strong leader who grappled with moments of personal internal fear and emotional discomfort; and (2) the heightened sense of racial identity during quarantine.

Theme One: The Strong Woman In-charge is Depressed and Scared and Exhausted

I must first acknowledge that I am a middle-aged single woman "sandwiched" between an aging parent and three young adult children. This term was first coined by social worker Dorothy Miller, originally in 1981, to describe women in their thirties to forties who were "sandwiched" between young children and aging parents as their primary caregiver (419). According to Parker and

Patten's (2013), 47% of adults in their forties and fifties are caring for an adult sixty-five or older while raising a young child or supporting a grown child (1). The authors assert that life in the sandwich generation could be a bit stressful. Living with an aging parent while still raising or supporting one's own children presents certain challenges not faced by other adults, such as caregiving and providing emotional support to both parent and children (Parker and Patten 2013, 4). Additionally, research has shown that the increased responsibility that comes with being a sandwich generation caregiver can lead to negative effects on caregivers' overall well-being (Remennick 1999, 347). These women reported that increased caregiving burden led to chronic fatigue, reduced social integration, and poor health habits (Remennick 1999, 350). Boyczuk and Fletcher (2015) found that sandwich generation women reported being overwhelmed, and had more on their plate than they could handle (52).

The pandemic also significantly increased the stress for caregivers and those of the sandwich generation, especially during quarantine. There were several reasons why stress increased for these populations, including threats to mortality, and disruptions to daily life such as social distancing and lockdown measures used to prevent the spread of infection (Artcher et al. 2021, 3).

My experiences align with the research above. I often felt stressed and burned out and that feeling has only been exacerbated during the COVID-19 pandemic. When the country went on "lockdown" and adopted a safer at home policy, I ended up sheltering in place with my three young adult children and my eighty-two-year-old father. This experience impacted me physically, mentally, emotionally, and ideologically. I often felt like I was negotiating my identity with myself and my family members. I was constantly asking myself who am I and what role should I take on? For instance, my father had been living with me for more than a year before the pandemic hit. Although I was his primary caregiver, I also had outside support and help from hired caregivers. To limit the amount of people my dad came in contact with, I had to temporarily suspend his physical therapy and companion care because I wanted to mitigate his exposure to the virus. Although I thought our relationship was the same, my father's view of our relationship had shifted as I assumed all of the caregiving roles. He now saw me as his caregiver, nurse, maid, cook, and companion. In addition to the stress brought on by being his sole caregiver, I was also saddened by this ideological shift. I just wanted to be his daughter. My father was no longer the person who could rescue me from life's challenges, instead he was now expecting me to be his source of comfort and well-being.

My children, on the other hand, brought on other identity issues that I chronicle in my narratives. Although I adore my children, as a single parent I could not wait for them to 'grow up' (which for me was turning eighteen and going to college). I thought that they were capable of taking care of themselves, not necessarily financially, but I thought they could take care of laundry and household chores. When my sons came home to quarantine, they resorted to their nine and eleven-year-old selves waiting for mom to take care of them. There seemed to be a disconnect between who I thought I should be to them and how they perceived my role as their mother. I saw myself as an adult living with four other capable adults who could help me during this time. I thought everyone could and should help with all of the household chores. My family members, however, saw me as *the* sole source of comfort and strength and as the person who was responsible for taking care of them. I constantly had to communicate my identity to them. I had to reiterate that although I was still their mother, they were grown and they should assume some of the household responsibilities. I was okay with being the leader of the team but I needed everyone on the team to work together.

Finally, instead of just being their mom I had to become the "COVID" police and gatekeeper. My children were no different than other young adults of similar ages who didn't take the virus seriously. While they were not going to crowded parties where attendees refused to social distance or wear masks, they refused to shelter in place with our five family members. Every other day someone who wasn't part of my immediate family would come over. When I discovered that my children had friends over, I would have a private conversation with them and explain that we should not have company in our home. In response they often said, "We are not going to be in the common areas. We will stay in my room away from you and Papa." I resented that I had to constantly play the role as the mean mom or bad guy. I just wanted to enjoy this time with my children. In addition to my fluctuating identities that I experienced with my father and children, I experienced a heightened sense of racial identity during the COVID-19 Crisis.

Theme Two: Racial Identity

I have always been aware of my "Blackness," and being Black has had both positive and negative impacts on my identity. For instance, when I didn't get a job or a promotion, I often wondered if my race played a role in being left out or looked over. When I was a younger woman, I worked as an entry-level interviewer at an insurance company. One time I passed a Black male prospective hire to the next level, and he was not hired. When I questioned the manager as to why the man wasn't hired, he responded by saying I want someone who is exceptional. On paper this man was exceptional, and he had excellent interpersonal skills and previous sales experience. We later hired someone who was an average white male. This gentleman was let go a year later. I have also had positive experiences where I've embraced my identity as a Black woman and have been proud for notable Black accomplishments. For instance, when someone Black becomes the "first" to complete a monumental achievement, such as Barack Obama becoming the first Black president, and most recently when Kamala Harris became the first Black female vice president. Although I am very aware of my identity as a Black woman, there are times when I feel a deeper connection to being Black. Quarantine was one of those times where I felt a heightened sense of my racial identity.

My identity was impacted for two reasons. One reason was that African Americans were impacted by COVID-19 at a disproportionate rate at the beginning of the pandemic (Reyes 2020, 299) According to Nemo (2020, 1), in Chicago, where African Americans comprise a third of the city's population, they account for half of those who have tested positive for the coronavirus, and almost three-quarters of COVID-19 deaths (1). Likewise, in Milwaukee County, Wisconsin, African Americans make up 70% of deaths due to the coronavirus, but just 26% of the county's population (1). In Louisiana, roughly 70% of those who have died of COVID-19 are African American, yet African Americans make up only 32.2% of the state's population (1). The disproportion is similar in Michigan: 33% of the COVID-19 cases and 40% of COVID-19-related deaths have been among African Americans, but African Americans comprise only 14% of the state's population (1). Wilkes (2020) states that 1–1,000 African Americans have died from COVID-19 (1). In December 2020, the cases that reported race and ethnicity indicated that African Americans account for 13.4 (CDC 2021), however, according to the U.S. Census Bureau, Black Non-Hispanic African Americans are only 12% of the total U.S. population. Although Black people are minorities in the country, the incidents and the deaths are higher than their white counterparts, at least at the start of the pandemic. The high numbers were alarming and very scary for me.

The second reason I had a heightened sense of racial identity was because of the number of racially motivated shootings that took place during quarantine. The deaths of Brianna Taylor, George Floyd, and Ahmaud Arbery occurred at the height of the pandemic while we were sheltering in place. The incidents sparked peaceful protests and a resurgence of the Black Lives Matter (BLM) movement around the world. These incidents were televised, and the videoclips were shown on all of the networks repeatedly. In the past when I heard about other similar incidents, I used to shrug it off as something that couldn't happen to me or my children. I told myself that the impacted individuals had prior lengthy records or other factors that led to their killings, like resisting arrest. However, while in quarantine I identified with the victims and I became fearful. Ahmuad Arbery was on a daily run in his neighborhood and was shot by his neighbors (Light and Thomas 2020, 1). Brianna was asleep in her bed when the police stormed into her apartment and killed her (Callimachi 2020, 2.). These incidents reminded me of what it means to be Black in the United States. According to Davis et. al., (2020) African American women live in neighborhoods with longstanding legacies of disinvestment and neglect. This lack in community funding ultimately results in neighborhoods that are deemed to be run down and hazardous (917). Knowing this, I have made a conscious effort to live in areas that are deemed safe (i.e., the suburbs). Most of the time I feel safe because I thought I took the necessary steps to protect myself and my children from such brutality (i.e., I got an education, I am gainfully employed and I moved into a safe neighborhood). Watching these incidents on television during quarantine changed my identity from a mom living in the safe suburbs, to a constantly fearful mom who is always on guard due to the color of my skin. I'm not sure if I will ever be the same.

Although much has been written in the literature about what it means to be Black in America, scholarship has begun to emerge discussing being Black during dual pandemics (meaning COVID-19 and racial violence). Lipscom and Ashley (2020), discuss how the mental health of Black individuals has suffered due to the pandemic. The authors describe the emotional labor of racialization, constantly navigating stereotypes, implicit bias and ongoing oppression as heavy (231). Additionally, the authors note that managing this heaviness juxtaposed with the virus, the isolation of quarantine, and the media portrayals of multiple murders as heavy and "soul wounding" (231). David Stamps (2020), who is also the parent of two Black sons, shares the sentiment of worrying about how this time in our country (the pandemic and racial unrest) will impact his sons emotional and physical health (134). The author also acknowledges the intersectionality of his role as a parent, and as a Black person, researcher, teacher and activist and that these identities cannot be compartmentalized (134). In the upcoming months and years, I am sure similar research will emerge as Black scholars record their experiences during these crises. I found the articles both sad and encouraging. I was sad to know that others were feeling that same way however, I was encouraged to know that I wasn't the only Black scholar and parent feeling overwhelmed and traumatized.

CONCLUDING THOUGHTS

It's been a year since my children and I sheltered in place together. In many ways our life has resumed some form of normalcy. My sons, for example, have returned to college, and my daughter has returned to high school. A year ago, I felt like I was living in a fishbowl, and we were always bumping into each other. Living in close quarters with four other people (my three children and my dad) whom I considered adults, was difficult at times. I learned a lot about myself, my father, and my children. There was often conflict between who my family expected me to be, and who I wanted to be in my role as mother and caregiver. Using the lens of CTI, there was a conflict between my enacted identity (which is my identity that is performed or expressed) and my relational identity (which is how I identified myself through my relationships with others) (Jung and Hecht 2005, 266). Montgomery and Kosloski (2009), acknowledge "caregiving as a process of changing identity" (48). The authors state that the caregiving role emerges out of existing role relationships such as daughter or wife (48.) Over time, as the recipients' needs change, the caregiver changes behaviors, and they also change the way they see their role (49). According to Montgomery and Kosloski (2009), those changes impact the way caregivers see themselves, resulting in a change of identity (49). Quarantine really intensified this change in my role as my father's caregiver, versus my identity as "his baby girl."

I have now made peace with the fact that those days will never return and my dad needs me to help take care of him. Living with my children during quarantine was a completely different story. I realized that I needed to set boundaries and communicate to them that although I was their mom, we are all adults and everyone is capable of doing their part. Now, I have started communicating my expectations clearly to all of my family members, and they have changed their behavior. As far as my racial identity, some of my fears have begun to subside, and I'm not as obsessed about dying from the virus or that my sons will be shot by the police. Although I know both are possibilities, I have made a conscious choice to be mindful and cautious. However, I have begun to be hopeful and to think positively about all of our futures. I have also learned to embrace every aspect of my identity (caregiver, mom, proud Black woman, and once in a while, superwoman) realizing that none of these identities cannot be compartmentalized—they are all me.

REFERENCES

APM Research Lab Staff. 2020. "The Color of Coronavirus: COVID-19 Deaths by Race and Ethnicity in the U.S." Accessed April 1, 2021. https://www.apmresearchlab.org/COVID/deaths-by-race.

Appold, Karen. 2020. "Deadly and revealing toll COVID-19 Has Taken on The African American Community." Accessed April 1, 2021. https://www.managedhealthcareexecutive.com/view/deadly-and-revealing-toll-covid-19-has-taken-african-american-community.

Archer, Jessie, Wendy Reiboldt, Maria Claver and John Fay. 2021. "Caregiving in Quarantine: Evaluating the Impact of the Covid-19 Pandemic on Adult Child Informal Caregivers of a Parent." *Gerontology & Geriatric Medicine,* 7: 1–7.

Boyczuk, Alana M. and Paula C. Fletcher. 2016. "The Ebbs and Flows: Stresses of Sandwich Generation Caregivers." *Journal of Adult Development,* 23, no. 1: 51–61.

Buttell, Frederick, Clare E.B. Cannon, Katherine Rose, and Regardt J. Ferreira. 2021. "COVID-19 and Intimate Partner Violence: Prevalence of Resilience and Perceived Stress During a Pandemic." *Traumatology.* http://dx.doi.org/10.1037/trm0000296.

Callimachi, Rukmini. 2020. "Breonna Taylor's Life Was Changing. Then the Police Came to Her Door." *The New York Times,* August 30, 2020. https://www.nytimes.com/2020/08/30/us/breonna-taylor-police-killing.html.

"COVID-19 Racial and Ethnic Health Disparities." Accessed March 26, 2021. https://www.cdc.gov/coronavirus/2019-ncov/community/health-equity/racial-ethnic-disparities/disparities-deaths.html.

Denyvetta Davis, Cheree Harris, Venita Johnson, Cheryl Pennington, Cresha Redus, Tiffani Sanders, Net-Hetep Ta-Nesert, Gina Sofola, Vanessa Morrison, John Harris and Eyakem Gulilat. 2020. "Black women's perspectives on neighborhood safety: Reflections from The Women of Northeast Oklahoma City Photovoice Project." *Gender, Place & Culture,* 27, no. 7: 917–943, www.https://doi.org/10.1080/0966369X.2019.1611547.

Ellis, Carolyn, Tony E. Adams, and Arthur Bochner. 2011. "Autoethnography: An Overview". *Forum: Qualitative Social Research,* 12, no. 1, Article 10. https://www.qualitative-research.net/index.php/fqs/article/view/1589/3095.

Ellis, Carolyn and Arthur, P. Bochner. 2000. "Autoethnography, Personal Narrative, Reflexivity. In *Handbook of Qualitative Research* (2nd Ed.), edited by Norman K. Denzin and Yvonna S. Lincoln, 733–768. Thousand Oaks: Sage.

Hecht, Michael L., Jennifer R. Warren, Eura Jung, and Janice Krieger. 2005. "The Communication Theory of Identity: Development, Theoretical Perspective, and Future Directions." In *Theorizing and Intercultural Communication,* edited by William B. Gudykunst, 259. Thousand Oaks: Sage.

Golden, Sherita, Hill. 2020. "Coronavirus in African Americans and Other People of Color." Accessed April 1, 2020, https://www.hopkinsmedicine.org/health/conditions-and-diseases/coronavirus/covid19-racial-disparities.

Jung, Eura, and Hecht, Michael L. 2004. "Elaborating the Communication Theory of Identity: Identity Gaps and Communication Outcomes." *Communication Quarterly,* 52 no. 33: 265–283.

Karimi, Faith and Maggie, Fox. 2020. "George Floyd Tested Positive for Coronavirus but it Had Nothing to Do with His Death Autopsy Shows." *CNN,* June 4, 2020. https://www.cnn.com/2020/06/04/health/george-floyd-coronavirus-autopsy/index.html.

Kim, Sage J. and Wendy Bostwick. 2020. "Social Vulnerability and Racial Inequality in COVID-19 Deaths in Chicago." *Health Education & Behavior,* 47, no. 4: 509–513. www.https://doi.org/10.1177/1090198120929677external icon.

Light, Caroline, and Janae Thomas. 2020. "Ahmaud Arbery was killed, allegedly by vigilantes. Racism Allowed Them to Claim Self-Defense." *The Washington Post,*

May 8, 2020. https://www.washingtonpost.com/outlook/2020/05/08/ahmaud-arbery-video-arrest/.

Lipscom, Allen E., and Wendy Ashley. 2020. "Surviving Being Black and a Clinician During a Dual Pandemic: Personal and Professional Challenges in a Disease and Racial Crisis." *Smith College Studies in Social Work*, 90, no. 4: 222–236. www.https://doi.org/10.1080/00377317.2020.1834489.

Mental health and Coping With Stress." 2021. Accessed April 1, 2021. https://www.cdc.gov/coronavirus/2019-ncov/daily-life-coping/managing-stress-anxiety.html.

Miller, Dorothy A. 1981."The Sandwich Generation: The Adult Children of The Aging. Social Work." *Social Work,* 26, no. 5: 419–423. https://doi.org/10.1093/sw/26.5.419.

Montgomery Rhonda, and Karl Kosloski. 2009. "Caregiving as a Process of Changing Identity: Implications For Caregiver Support." *Generations,* 33, no. 1: 47–52.

Nemo, Leslie. 2020. "Why People of Color Are Disproportionately Hit by COVID-19" *Discover Magazine*. https://www.discovermagazine.com/health/why-people-of-color-are-disproportionately-hit-by-covid-19.

"Quick Facts: United States." 2020. *The United States Census Bureau.* Accessed April 1, 2020. https://www.census.gov/quickfacts/fact/table/US/PST045219.

Remennick, Larissa I. (1999). "Women of the 'Sandwich' Generation and Multiple Roles: The case of Russian Immigrants of the 1990s in Israel." *Sex Roles*, 40, no: 5/6: 347–378.

Scott, Eugene. "Four Reasons Coronavirus is hitting Black Communities so Hard." 2020. *The Washington Post,* April 10, 2020. https://www.washingtonpost.com/politics/2020/04/10/4-reasons-coronavirus-is-hitting- Black-communities-so-hard/.

Stamps, David. 2021. "The Collective Challenges of Color, COVID-19, and Their Convergence." *Journal of Children and Media*, 15, no. 1: 134–137. www.https://doi.org/10.1080/17482798.2020.1858903.

Taratine, Ruth. 2014. "The Sandwich Generation: Who is Caring for You?" *The Huffington Post,* September 7, 2014. https://www.huffpost.com/entry/baby-boomers-caregivers_b_5733782.

Wagner, P. 2017. "Bulking Up (Identities): A Communication Framework for Male Fitness Identity." *Communication Quarterly*, 64, no. 5: 580–602. https://doi.org/10.1080/01463373.2017.1321027.

Wilkes, Sybil. 2020. "Coronavirus Update: 1 in 1,000 African Americans Have Died from Coronavirus." *Black America Web.* Accessed April 1, 2021. https://Blackamericaweb.com/2020/10/01/coronavirus-update-1-in-1000-african-americans-have-died-from-coronavirus/.

Part II

MASS COMMUNICATION

Chapter 3

Sports Diplomacy in the Age of the COVID-19 Pandemic

Katherine Loh

The World Health Organization (WHO) continues to track the progression of COVID-19 as it treks a deadly path through countries. The COVID-19 timeline tells a story of a virus that is methodical, precise, and tenacious in its objective—survival. In its path, COVID-19 has left behind tattered economies, shattered communities, and death. The virus was first recorded on the WHO timeline on December 31, 2019, as a "viral pneumonia" case in Wuhan, China (WHO 2020, par. 1). By January 9, 2020, Chinese authorities had determined that the outbreak was caused by a novel coronavirus, with the first reported death in China recorded on January 11, 2020 (WHO 2020, par. 1).

The virus arrived on U.S. soil on January 21, 2020, and was detected in France on January 24, 2020. Within a span of days, the virus was recorded in three continents. The WHO issued an advisory to the public on mask wearing as a means to mitigate the risk of catching the virus as early as January 2020 (WHO 2020). COVID-19 received its official name on February 11, 2020, and in the same month, the virus made its way to the African continent (WHO 2020). On March 11, 2020, the WHO declared COVID-19 a global pandemic (WHO 2020) and the world as we have grown to know it, changed forever.

As the world struggled to understand and ultimately manage the virus, governments and local officials failed to come up with comprehensive plans to mitigate the spread. School closures led to business closures, which led to lockdowns of entire cities and countries. Infection and death rates continued to rise as the WHO reported over 1 million confirmed cases of infection worldwide by April of 2020 (WHO 2020). The effects of the virus were not felt equally by all countries and communities. Some were more impacted than others, but one group in particular truly felt the full brunt of COVID-19.

COVID-19 AND ITS BLIGHT ON NATIVE AMERICAN COMMUNITIES

According to the Center for Disease Control (CDC): "American Indian and Alaska Native persons appear to be disproportionately affected by the COVID-19 pandemic" (Hatcher et al. 2020, 1). This effect can be attributed to a long history of inadequate health care infrastructure, poverty in some Native American communities, and a culture that revolves around multi-generational living. These factors, under the light of a pandemic, accelerated the spread of the virus (Hatcher et al. 2020, 1). The CDC study found Native Americans are 3.5 times more likely to contract COVID-19 than non-Hispanic white populations (Hatcher et al. 2020, par. 2; Reuters 2020, par. 2). In addition, COVID-19 has affected the younger population of Native Americans at a higher rate compared to non-Hispanic white populations: COVID-19 infected 12.9% of Native American youths while the infection rate of non-Hispanic white youths was 4.3% (Reuters 2020, par. 3). For example, in Montana, Native Americans make up 6.6% of the population, and hold 17% of the state's COVID-19 infection cases and 32% of COVID-19 deaths (Mabie 2020, par. 1). Furthermore, Native Americans in Montana are hospitalized as a result of COVID-19 at a rate of 12%, compared to the lower 7% rate of Montana's white population, while both infections and deaths are also concentrated in the Crow Nation communities (Mabie 2020, par. 1). These disparities can be traced to serious preexisting health conditions in the Native American population, a seriously underfunded health care system serving Native American communities, and crowded homes (multi-generational living) oftentimes coupled with subpar infrastructure such as plumbing (Ayesh 2020, par. 3–9). According to Stacey Bohlen, CEO of the National Indian Health Board: "Navajo Nation surpassed New York City for the highest COVID-19 infection rate." (Frieden 2020, par. 5). The disparities are stark and they are sobering: "If tribes were states, the top five infection rates nationwide would be tribal nations" (Frieden 2020, par. 5). In the midst of such a public health crisis, how can one communicate health information effectively to the most vulnerable of communities?

STRATEGIC COMMUNICATION AND SPORTS DIPLOMACY

Strategic Communication is defined as "the purposeful use of communication by an organization to fulfill its mission" (Hallahan et al. 2007, 3). At the core of strategic communication, organizations, or individuals, who are adept at this skillset, understand that it is multidisciplinary in nature—pulling from multiple methods and subject areas in communication (Hallahan et al. 2007, 3). According to Vaughan and Tinker (2009) effective strategic communication during a public health crisis, especially when vulnerable communities or groups are concerned, is not only essential, but it is critical to the success of health risk communication (Vaughan & Tinker 2009, S324). They argue that at the crux of these strategic communication efforts lies *trust* which can occur when health risk communication messages are catered to target a community's culture, language, and life conditions. They also note that utilizing an appropriate spokesperson to deliver health messages in empathetic ways can also build trust (Vaughan & Tinker 2009, S372; Reddy & Gupta 2020, 3795; Schiavo 2020, 74).

Sports Diplomacy is understood as a deliberate and strategic deployment of athletes or athletic events as tools for states to achieve various objectives (Murray 2018). Sports, and the athletes we look up to, "can be thought of as a form of diplomacy in its own right. It transcends politics, unites strangers through a common, anthropological love of games, and as such, is one of the great civil, civilised and civilising institutions" (Murray 2018, 53). In other words, the world we live in is equally influenced by formally appointed Sports Diplomats as we are by the informal Sports Diplomat we idolize. As such, a Sports Diplomat exhibits many qualities. While their role can be formal or informal, Sports Diplomats are first and foremost recognized as highly accomplished in their sport, demonstrate an ability to use their voice and representation over various social justice issues, are visible and vocal on social media, and have an established relationship with their fan base (Loh 2020, 92–99; Pigman 2014, 2; Wahl 2019, par. 9; Vanc 2013, 1190).

Strategic Communication and Sports Diplomacy is a potent partnership, especially if the athlete understands the power of social media and the "weaponization" of the various platforms in their messaging objectives (Loh, 2020, 91). As Freberg (2019) stated, "the sports industry and social media have become integrated" (243) and "when exploring how to apply social media, one field that constantly pushes the envelope for innovation and creativity is the sports industry" (243).

From a strategic communication perspective, athletes use social media around the following themes: presenting themselves as role models, bringing awareness to important issues, helping others, establishing their presence through engagement or endorsements, branding, and entertaining (Freberg 2019, 243–245). From a Sports Diplomacy perspective, athletes tend to be very effective in communicating issues related to human security, including pandemic and public health (Murray 2018, 169). Athletes, and in particular, athletes who also inhabit the Sports Diplomat role, can do this because they are viewed as authentic, relatable, credible, believable, genuine, charitable, and heroic (Murray 2018, 170–173). Their fans and the public tend to trust them more than they would a politician or a state-affiliated diplomat because their status as a hero is connected to the narrative that they are like us: they too can fail. "We trust sportspeople as communicators, for they are us" (Murray 2018, 173). When Sports Diplomats communicate strategically via social media, they have the ability to "amplify and spread" (Murray 2018, 106) messages and when those messages are related to issues of human security, such as a global pandemic, the effects can be powerful.

SPORTS IN A PANDEMIC

The declaration of COVID-19 as a global pandemic impacted every sector of every country. One particular aspect of COVID-19 that intersects with economic, political, and societal impacts is sports. As countries went into quarantine and lockdowns, sports leagues canceled or postponed major competitions. From youth recreational programs to major Olympic events, the sounds of competition went silent in 2020.

In the United States and in particular collegiate sports, the spring sports season of 2020 was particularly gut-wrenching for the student-athletes. On March 12, 2020, the National Collegiate Athletics Association (NCAA) announced all winter and spring sports canceled for the rest of the year. Eventually, colleges moved to shut down and students sent home to continue their classes remotely. For all graduating winter and spring collegiate athletes, COVID-19 was a season-ending event not caused by an injury (DaSilva 2020; NCAA 2020).

As the pandemic prevailed through the summer, colleges and universities implemented very different return to school and return to play plans. But as 2020 drew to a close, the world saw the Tokyo Olympics postponed to 2021, the NCAA canceled fall and winter sports, and World Lacrosse postponed two World Championships scheduled for 2021 to 2022. The "financial Armageddon" of missed revenues from canceled or postponed events were felt by event organizers, institutions, and global economies. In college sports, one of the first victims of not playing one season of revenue-generating collegiate sports was Furman University Men's Lacrosse program, which was cut in the early summer of 2020 (Barrister 2020, par. 21).

Since it is a spring sport, lacrosse was severely impacted by COVID-19. In addition, as mentioned previously, COVID-19 has disproportionately affected Native American communities. Thus, since lacrosse originated in Native American tribes and Lyle Thompson is lacrosse's most recognized Sports Diplomat (Loh, 2020), this chapter will focus on lacrosse and Lyle Thompson. More specifically, this chapter will use a case study analysis to examine Sports Diplomacy in the time of pandemic within a community that is disproportionately impacted by COVID-19.

METHODOLOGY

Research Design

A case study analysis, defined as "a qualitative approach in which the investigator explores a real-life, contemporary bounded system" such as a case or multiple cases, "over time, through detailed, in-depth data collection involving multiple sources of information" (Creswell & Poth 2018, 96) was used in the current research study. More specifically, the current study used the single instrumental case study, in which "the researcher focuses on an issue or concern and then selects one bounded case to illustrate this issue" (Creswell & Poth 2018, 98).

As alluded to in previous sections of this chapter, Lyle Thompson fits the model of a Sports Diplomat, not only in the lacrosse world but also within his Native American community. He is active on social media and uses his social media platforms to communicate his thoughts on various issues to his fans. Thus, this research design falls within the parameters of a bounded case study (Creswell & Poth 2018, 100).

Facebook continues to rank as the dominant social media platform with about 2.5 billion active users as of April 2020 (Clement 2020, par. 1), and according to Clement's (2020) ranking report, Twitter was ranked in fourteenth place with about 366 million active users. The decision to use Twitter for this study was primarily driven by Twitter's unique communication design: "Twitter is designed to elicit frequent, unprompted, spontaneous, and unfiltered thoughts from its users, who come into conflict with one another as in no other medium, sometimes tweeting things they quickly regret" (Friedersdorf 2018, 1). It is exactly this raw and brutally honest nature of Twitter that makes it an ideal platform to access study subjects and their thoughts for thematic analysis.

Procedure and Data Analysis

This study tracked the Twitter feed of Lyle Thompson over a six-month period. During the same six-month period, interviews and articles about Lyle Thompson were also reviewed. Data pulled from these sources were used for thematic analysis.

Lyle Thompson's Twitter feed was tracked and analyzed from January 21, 2020, the date that the WHO recorded the first case of COVID-19 on U.S. soil (WHO 2020, par. 2), to July 21, 2020. The researcher tallied the number of original Tweets, number of re-Tweets, placed the Tweets into categories, and when the subject tweeted about COVID-19 or COVID-19 related content, the researcher would conduct a further thematic analysis of that content. During the same six-month period, the researcher also reviewed interviews and articles related to, and about Lyle Thompson. Articles and interviews specific to the pandemic were flagged and analyzed for themes.

RESULTS

In the six-month period of analysis, Lyle Thompson recorded a total of fifty-eight Tweets. From this total, thirty were re-Tweets and twenty-eight were unique Tweets. The Tweets were categorized and summarized into the following table:

Table 3.1 Summary of Lyle Thompson's Twitter Activity from January 21, 2020, through July 21, 2020

Category	Unique Tweets	Re-Tweets
Lacrosse Related	7	19
Health Related	5	0
Family Centered	1	1
Politics/Activism	0	4
Sports Related (not lacrosse)	5	3
Brand/Product Endorsements	7	2
Other (random photos)	2	1
COVID-19	1	0
TOTAL	28	30

In looking at the various topics where Thompson either generated an original Tweet, or re-Tweeted content from another source, it is evident that COVID-19 was *not* the focus of communication during the analysis period. The primary focus of communication was still lacrosse and lacrosse-related content, followed by sports-related content and brand and product-related/endorsement content. Thompson did not comment directly on content related to politics or activism, but instead, re-Tweeted content from other sources (@gobidesert25, July 12, 2020; @IRQ_Nationals, July 18, 2020).

Thompson sent one Tweet on the issue of COVID-19 on April 11, 2020, in the format of a video message (See Appendix A for transcript). The video was two minutes and thirteen seconds in length and specifically addressed the impact of COVID-19 on the Native American community and what Native Americans, specifically the younger generation, could do about curbing the spread of the virus. In the video, Thompson addressed his fans, but more specifically the Native American community directly. His message was very genuine and personal, saying "I don't have the answers" as to why COVID-19 is hitting Native American communities especially hard (@lyle4thompson, April 11, 2020). He highlighted some of the reasons why COVID-19 spread more rapidly in Native American communities, as alluded to in previous paragraphs (e.g., multigenerational living) and reinforced CDC recommendations of social distancing, handwashing, and staying home. His message was also specific to the younger generation as a call to action, for them to be aware of their responsibility to take care of the more vulnerable members of their community (@lyle4thompson, April 11, 2020). Thompson started his message by emphasizing his lacrosse credentials "I'm a professional lacrosse player, N7 Ambassador, Nike Athlete" (@lyle4thompson, April 11, 2020) in which he clearly established his role as a Sports Diplomat. It should be noted that he posted a video and was able to speak at length about his thoughts about COVID-19 and worked around the 280-character limit of Twitter. Posting a video also allowed fans to see his nonverbal communication, which in this case, added to the authenticity and sincerity of the message. Finally, it is interesting to note that in the six-month period of review, Thompson posted only one time about COVID-19 (or any COVID-19 and pandemic-related topics). Given the severity of COVID-19 on Native American communities (Mabie 2020), and what we know about the importance of repeated and sustained public health messaging in order to be effective (Vaughan & Tinker 2009), it is of note that Thompson only commented on the matter once. An interview with the subject would yield further explanation to this observation but this was not part of the research design for this study.

In the six-month time frame of analysis there were two interviews Lyle Thompson conducted that touched on COVID-19 (LoRe 2020; Wang 2020). Information from these articles were also used for thematic analysis. In the articles, the subject talked about having a sense of lost identity when lacrosse ended due to COVID-19. He talked about the challenges of quarantine, figuring out what to do with all the free time in his hands, staying in shape, keeping his family safe, and still being able to compete at an elite level (LoRe 2020, par. 13–15). His concerns around the virus were summed up in this quote: "I know I am going to be battling against someone who I hope is taking those same precautions" (Wang 2020, par. 21). These concerns seem to mirror how Native American communities felt as they battled COVID-19 in their communities and their lack of control over the pandemic. Both articles echoed similar sentiments from Lyle and reiterated his concern for COVID-19 and his commitment to staying in shape and getting to play again (LoRe 2020, Wang 2020). While the articles do address and mention behaviors that will help curb the spread of COVID-19 (social distancing, wearing a mask), they cannot be perceived as public health messages. At best, one can only infer that fans of Thompson will read the interviews and emulate the public health behaviors described in the interview.

DISCUSSION

Thematic Analysis I: Expectations Placed on the Sports Diplomat

A holistic analysis approach was used to analyze content from Thompson's Twitter feed and available articles within the six-month period (Creswell & Poth, page 100).

Prior research suggests that the Native American community experienced more stressors due to COVID-19 than other communities (Hatcher et al. 2020). Even though there is an expectation that athletes who inhabit the role of a Sports Diplomat within a community also have a social responsibility to share public health information with their community (Murray 2018, 169), the data, in the case of Lyle Thompson, revealed a complexity to this perception. Of the fifty-eight Tweets, only one dealt with the pandemic, and in the six-month period, only two articles/interviews referenced the subject's views on the pandemic. Of all three references, only one Tweet specifically addressed COVID-19 directly as a public health issue for the Native American community and was used as a direct call to action to act responsibly for the greater good of the community.

There is a public expectation of Sports Diplomats to conduct and behave themselves in a certain way. In a socially mediated world, that expectation often also includes how frequent a Sports Diplomat posts about a particular topic. Not posting enough on COVID-19 may make the public perceive Thompson as insensitive or apathetic. Posting too much may suggest an air of inauthenticity. The Sports Diplomat simply cannot win because there is no equation or algorithm as to what is the appropriate amount to post. Expectation Dissonance (Loh 2021), a theory proposed in this study to help us understand this phenomenon, occurs when there is conflict between public expectation and actual strategic communication behavior of a Sports Diplomat around a distinct social issue. There is an expectation for Thompson, given his status as a high-profile Native American lacrosse player and Sports Diplomat, to be more vocal regarding COVID-19, considering how the pandemic is disproportionately affecting Native American communities. The analysis of the subject's Twitter feed showed the opposite to be true. From a social media context, there was Expectation Dissonance. Specifically, in the example of a public health crisis, one can argue that when there is an Expectation Dissonance (Sports Diplomat is not communicating to the expectation of the public around a distinct social issue) the consequences can be dire. In the case of Lyle Thompson, there was no discernable backlash that he did not speak up *enough* about the issue of COVID-19 on the Native American communities. It is important to understand why this is the case, which leads to the second thematic analysis.

Thematic Analysis II: Sports Diplomats are Strategic Communicators

Sports Diplomats *are* strategic communicators who understand the "weaponization of Facebook, Twitter, Instagram, Live Streaming, YouTube, Podcasts, Live Stream on Facebook, and so much more" (Loh 2020, 91) can augment and disseminate their messaging and brand globally. The analysis of the Thompson's Twitter feed supports this theme. During the six-month period of analysis, Thompson continued to Tweet on lacrosse (twenty-six total Tweets); brand and product endorsements (nine total Tweets); health-related content (five total Tweets); and other sports-related content (eight total Tweets). As a prominent Native American lacrosse player, Thompson continued to be an ambassador for the sport, with lacrosse tracking the highest number of Tweets. This was followed closely by product and brand-related content, as Thompson is also one of few lacrosse players who are highly sought after by brands for endorsements.

The data suggest that Sports Diplomats are very self-aware, that even in times of a pandemic, they are first and foremost an ambassador of their sport and if they have product endorsements, an ambassador for those products and brands. The subject continued to be focused on what his "diplomatic" responsibilities are: to his sports and his brand. Strategically, he managed his communication according to those responsibilities. Expectation Management (Loh 2021), as proposed by this researcher, is when a Sports Diplomat uses strategic communication to balance messaging responsibilities between distinct stakeholders and social issues.

In the analysis of Thompson's Tweets and interviews, he raised awareness of the issues around COVID-19 (e.g., impact on Native American communities, need to quarantine, encourage hand washing, social distance, and call for younger generations to take care of the older generations) (@lyle4thompson, April 11, 2020) and continued to be a role model to his many fans (e.g., portraying a positive attitude, sending many messages of staying fit, humorous and light-hearted content) (@lyle4thompson, March 23, 2020; April 10, 2020; May 6, 2020). Thompson maintained a presence with his fan base by calling on his fans to make a difference through helping others, continued to brand himself and the products who support him, and also continued to advocate for the right of the Native American lacrosse National team to play as a sovereign nation. Sports Diplomats, in their communication, raise awareness of issues, are role models, maintain a presence on social media so that they stay engaged with their fans, encourage fans to make a difference and help others, communicate to monetize their brand, and communicate to entertain. Sports Diplomats, regardless of the public health situation we are in, will tend to organize their strategic communication around these general themes (Freberg 2019, 243–246). How a

Sports Diplomat adjusts their communication frequency within these general themes, during times of a global pandemic, can be understood and analyzed using the Expectation Dissonance and Expectation Management theories. In the case of Lyle Thompson, one can argue that his use of Expectation Management was able to curb the negativity Expectation Dissonance may have generated.

Ultimately, the intent of the case is also important. Understanding how Sports Diplomats who inhibit the privilege of voice and representation in communities hit hard by COVID-19 will be important to understand how we can leverage strategic communication and Sports Diplomats more effectively in the realm of public health communication.

LIMITATIONS AND FUTURE RESEARCH

The bounded case study limited the study to one Sports Diplomat, in one sport, over a six-month period of analysis. More Sports Diplomats should be studied, across more sports and over a longer period of time. Comparative analysis can also be drawn between different sports and different social media platforms. Comparative analysis can also be done looking at data drawn in time of crisis and out of crisis. The theories of Expectation Dissonance and Expectation Management that emerged from this study, should be evaluated further as well. This study is a promising start and further studies should add understanding on the complex role of the Sports Diplomat, and their relationship with strategic communication tactics, as experienced in a myriad of social contexts.

APPENDIX A: FURTHER READING

Transcript of Lyle Thompson's Twitter Post

Twitter Account: @lyle4thompson
April 11, 2020

Caption: #protectourelders #Alonetogether #COVID-19
Length: 2 minutes 13 seconds

Text:

"What's up everybody? Lyle Thompson here. I'm a professional lacrosse player, N7 Ambassador, Nike athlete.

I wanted to send out a message to our native communities regarding the COVID-19 and I had gotten a few messages from some friends that are concerned, stressed about why this is affecting our community so much and I don't have the answers, obviously there's a lot of research that still needs to be done and that are being figured out right now but I do know that within our communities, we have a lot of elders and a lot of our grandparents and our parents are still living all in one household and that makes it really easy for this to spread right inside your own household, let alone the whole community, so it's important for our younger generations to make sure we're following these safety precautions: practicing social distancing, staying at home, washing your hands, staying clean—because at the end of the day, you follow that criteria, you're literally saving lives, so that's important and I wanted to send out a message and make sure our youth, the younger generation, the one's my age that may be less affected by it—but at the end of the day, you can be a carrier and you can pass it on.

Let's not bring this into our communities, let's not be another bad statistic. Right now is a perfect time to reconnect with yourself, to reconnect with nature. We're all in this together and um—I mean look at—you also gotta think about how good of a break we're giving Mother Earth right now and consider all that and at the end of the day I want to make sure our communities are as safe as possible, and we're all a part of that."

REFERENCES

Ayesh, Rashaan. 2020. "Native Americans Struggle to Fight the Coronavirus." *Axios*, May 16, 2020. https://www.axios.com/native-americans-unprepared-coronavirus-pandemic-62659a0-e49b-4a1b-bbf8-5cf3bc1df53b-html.

Barrister, Eri. 2020. "COVID Challenges: College Lacrosse's Uncertain Immediate Future." *SBNation*, May 19, 2020. https://www.collegecrosse.com/2020/5/19/21247048/covid-challenges-college-lacrosses-uncertain-immediate-future-universities.

Clement, J. 2020. "Global social networks ranked by number of users 2020." *Statista*. April 24, 2020. www.statista.com/statistics/272014/global-social-networks-ranked-by-number-of-uers/.

Creswell, John W., and Poth, Cheryl N. 2018. *Qualitative Inquiry & Research Design: Choosing Among Five Approaches*. 4th ed. California: Sage Publications.

DaSilva, Matt. 2020. "Coronavirus (COVID-19) Updates Related to Lacrosse." *US Lacrosse Magazine,* March 11, 2020. https://www.uslaxmagazine.com/college/coronavirus-covid-19-updates-related-to-lacrosse.

Freberg, Karen. 2019. *Social Media for Strategic Communication: Creative Strategies and Research-Based Applications*. California: Sage Publications.

Frieden, Joyce. 2020. "Native Americans Need More Funding to Battle COVID-19, Lawmakers Told." *MedPage Today,* June 12, 2020. https://www.medpagetoday.com/infectiousdisease/covid19/87032.

Friedersdorf, Conor. 2018. "What Twitter still doesn't understand about its responsibility." *The Atlantic*, January 11, 2018. https://www.theatlantic.com/politics/archive/2018/01/at-least-nudge-world-leaders-to-tweet-responsibly/550013/.

Hallahan, Kirk, Holtzhausen Derina, van Ruler Betteke, Verčič Dejan, and Sriramesh Krishnamurthy. 2007. "Defining Strategic Communication." *International Journal of Strategic Communication* 1(1): 3–35. https://doi.org/10.1080/15531180701285244.

Hatcher, SM, Agnew-Brune C, Anderson M, et al. 2020. "COVID-19 Among American Indian and Alaska Native Persons - 23 States, January 31–July 3, 2020." *Morbidity and Mortality Weekly Report,* August 28, 2020, 69: 1166–1169. http://dx.doi.org/10.15585/mmwr.mm6934e1.

Loh, Katherine. 2020. "Sports Diplomacy and Conflict Framing: An Analysis of How Celebrity Athletes Influence Discourse in Race and Politics." in *The Role of Conflict on the Individual and Society*, edited by Theresa MacNeil-Kelly, 87–102, Lanham: Lexington Press.

Lore, Michael. 2020. "Lacrosse star Lyle Thompson is ready to resume play, but remains cautious." *Forbes*, May 21, 2020. https://www.forbes.com/sites/michaellore/2020/05/21/lacrosse-star-lyle-thompson-is-ready-to-resume-play-but-remains-cautious/#2cb7405735e8.

Mabie, Nora. 2020. "Native American tribes have been hit harder by COVID-19. Here's why." *Great Falls Tribune,* August 5, 2020. https://www.greatfallstribune.com/story/news/2020/08/05/why-native-americans-impacted-harder-covid-19-montana-united-states/5573737002/.

Murray, Stuart. 2018. *Sports Diplomacy: Origins, Theory and Practice.* New York: Routledge Press.

NCAA. 2020. "COVID-19 Coronavirus." http://www.ncaa.org/sport-science-institute/covid-19-coronavirus.

Pigman, Geoffrey Allen. "International Sport and Diplomacy's Public Dimension: Governments, Sporting Federations and the Global Audience." *Diplomacy & Statecraft* 25, no. 1 (February 2014): 94–114. https://doi.org/10.1080/09592296.2014.873613.

Reddy, B., and A. Gupta. 2020. "Importance of Effective Communication during COVID-19 Infodemic." *Journal of Family Medicine & Primary Care* 9(8): 3793–3796. https://doi.org/10.4103/jfmpc.jfmpc_719_20.

Reuters. 2020. "American Indians, Alaska Natives Hit Harder by COVID-19, U.S. CDC Says." *Reuters*, August 19, 2020. https://www.reuters.com/article/us-health-coronavirus-usa-race/american-indians-alaska-natives-hit-harder-by-covid-19-u-s-cdc-says-idUSKCN25F2KG.

Schiavo, R. 2020 "Vaccine Communication in the Age of COVID-19: Getting Ready for an Information War." *Journal of Communication in Healthcare* 13(2): 73–75. https://doi.org/10.1080/17538068.2020.1778959.

Thompson, Lyle (@lyle4thompson). 2020. Twitter, January 21 to July 21, 2020.

Vanc, Antoaneta M. 2013. "The Counter-Intuitive Value of Celebrity Athletes as Antidiplomats in Public Diplomacy: Ilie Nastase from Romania and the World of Tennis." *Sport in Society* 17(9): 1187–1203. https://doi.org/10.1080/17430437.2013.856591.

Vaughan, E., and T. Tinker. 2009. "Effective Health Risk Communication About Pandemic Influenza for Vulnerable Populations." *American Journal of Public Health* 99(S2): S324–S332. https://doi.org/10.2105/AJPH.2009.162537.

Wahl, Grant. "Megan Rapinoe Uses her FIFA Best Platform to Inspire." *Sports Illustrated*, September 23, 2019. https://www.si.com/soccer/2019/09/23/megan-rapinoe-fifa-best-player-award-speech.

Wang, Gene. 2020. "Lyle Thompson Stands up for Native American Heritage as Lacrosse Superstar." *The Washington Post*, July 15, 2020. https://www.washingtonpost.com/sports/2020/07/15/lyle-thompson-stands-up-native-american-heritage-lacrosse-superstar/.

World Health Organization. 2020. "Timeline of WHO's Response to COVID-19, last updated 30 July, 2020." https://who.int/news-room/detail/29-06-2020-covidtimeline.

Chapter 4

Agenda Setting

A Thematic Analysis of The New York Times *COVID-19 Coverage*

Theresa MacNeil-Kelly

The first case of the novel coronavirus (COVID-19) occurred in China in December 2019, with many reports originally tracing its genesis to a seafood and poultry market in Wuhan, China (Taylor 2021). However, more recent accounts refute this (Gorman and Barnes 2021), and as of March 30, 2021, The World Health Organization (WHO) reports that they are still investigating all hypotheses related to the origin of the virus (WHO 2021). Thus far, COVID-19 has killed more than 1.6 million individuals and has infected at least 76 million (Taylor 2021). On January 21, 2020, the Centers of Disease Control and Prevention (CDC) reported that the first case of travel-related COVID-19 was detected in the United States, and on March 11, 2020, the WHO declared COVID-19 a worldwide pandemic (WHO 2020). On March 15, 2020, the CDC recommended that people avoid gathering in groups of more than fifty people, which was around the same time that a considerable amount of states in the United States began to implement a stay-at-home or safer-at-home order, in an effort to slow the spread of COVID-19 (Taylor 2021).

According to agenda-setting theory, the agenda of the media becomes the prominent, salient, agenda for the public. In short, "the more coverage an issue receives, the more important it is to the people" (Coleman et al. 2009, 147). Because of the growing interest in and spreading of the virus and the increase of quarantine protocols in the United States during the months of March and April 2020 (Taylor 2021), several news outlets reported solely on COVID-19.

Thus, the purpose of this chapter is to understand, via thematic analysis, news media coverage in the United States in *The New York Times* during the early months (March 2020 and April 2020) of the COVID-19 virus spread in the United States. In order to make sense of the data, the present research used agenda-setting theory as a framework to understand emerging themes.

AGENDA-SETTING THEORY

The genesis of agenda-setting theory is credited to Lippmann's (1922) *Public Opinion,* which first suggested the media's power in shaping the opinions of an audience (317). Later, McCombs and Shaw (1972) tested the hypothesis in the 1968 presidential race between Hubert Humphrey and Richard Nixon, analyzing local and national media and comparing the media agenda to issues important to local voters (177). Their results yielded a high correlation between the agenda of the media and that of local voters, and agenda setting was born (185).

Subsequent research corroborated McCombs and Shaw's (1972) groundbreaking results.

For example, past research suggests that the public adopts the media's agenda in as little as five to seven weeks, and continues to find media topics salient even after coverage has ceased (Salwen 1988, 100). Moreover, agenda setting has been confirmed globally, "at national and local events, in elections and non-elections, with newspapers and television" (Coleman et al. 2009, 149).

This first concept of agenda theory has been termed "first level." According to Coleman et al. (2009), "whereas first level agenda setting focuses on the amount of media coverage an issue or other topic receives, the 'second level' of agenda setting looks at how the media discuss those issues or other objects of attention, such as public figures" (149). In other words, the way that the media describes public personas are similar to the public's perception of these individuals or salient issues (149). In sum, first-level agenda setting is most concerned with the influence of the media and which subjects are at the center of public attention, whereas second-level agenda setting is concerned with how individuals understand the ideas that have captured their attention (150).

METHODOLOGY

Sample

All articles in the sample came from *The New York Times* online newspaper archive database. *The New York Times* periodical was chosen over others because it provided the most amount of articles on COVID-19 and has been awarded the most journalism Pulitzer Prizes of any newspaper outlet (Nafria 2018). Selection of specific articles was determined by two mandates. First, articles had to be centered around the subject of COVID-19, and second, articles had to be written between March 1 and April 30, 2020. These dates were specifically chosen in order to get an overall understanding of material published during the first two months of the COVID-19 pandemic and to keep research results parsimonious and focused. Additionally, as mentioned previously, the coronavirus began spreading more rapidly in the United States during the months of March and April 2020, with many states moving to stay-at-home or safer-at-home directives (Taylor 2021), and therefore the sample focused on only these two months of news coverage.

Criterion sampling, which is used when specific criteria is needed to examine a sample (Miles and Huberman 1994, 28), was the primary means of extracting relevant articles. In the current study, criteria for stories were based on those that were in the "U.S." section, under "article" type of *The New York Times,* as well as those that included such terms as "virus," "pandemic," "Coronavirus," and "COVID-19." Identifying the articles involved first going to *The New York Times* website and searching the archive for all articles between March 1, 2020, and April 30, 2020. From this search, seventy-eight articles had connections to the relevant criteria search terms.

Data Analysis

A general thematic analysis was first conducted on the seventy-eight relevant news articles in order to extract common themes. According to Guest, MacQueen and Namey (2011), "thematic analyses move beyond counting explicit words or phrases and focus on identifying and describing both implicit and explicit ideas within the data, that is, themes" (10). Each article was read first holistically to get a clearer understanding of first-level agenda-setting ideas, and then was re-read a second time to look for more specific second-level agenda setting thematic elements. During each read, notes were taken and emerging themes were discovered from the ideas in the articles.

RESULTS

Using first-level and second-level agenda setting to analyze seventy-eight salient articles in *The New York Times,* three themes were extracted that received abundant news coverage within the span of March 1, 2020, to April 30, 2020. These included dread, mitigation, and the economy.

Dread

Dread was a common theme throughout the news coverage in *The New York Times* during March 2020 and April 2020. Coverage included several repetitive dire words and phrases such as "death," "worse-case scenario," and "suffering." On April 1, *The Times* noted that The United Nations secretary general, Antonio Guterres, called the coronavirus the biggest threat to humanity since World War II (Lyons 2020, April 1, 2020), and then later reported that because of the virus, the world was in the worst economy since the Great Depression (Lyons 2020, April 1, 2020). In the month of March 2020, reports of Wall Street plunging, events being canceled, like concerts, and sports seasons such as basketball, baseball, and hockey, took precedence in the news coverage (Lyons 2020, March 12, 2021). This same month reports about increases of sickness in not just older people, but younger individuals, like millennials, and lack of ventilators across the globe (Lyons 2020, March 18, 2021) were also prevalent stories. Other stories that elicited dread included the mention of the WHO declaring a pandemic and travel changes, including the closing of the Mexican/U.S. and Canadian/U.S. borders, as well as travel bans for European Union (EU) and Chinese citizens coming to the United States (Lyons 2020, March 12, 2021).

News coverage focused on hypothetical elements also incited dread. For instance, in a March 13 article, *The New York Times* reported that President Trump had declared a national emergency due to the rising cases in the United States, climbing to almost 2,000 and the death toll increasing to forty-one (*The New York Times* 2020, March 13, 2020). Due to this, *The Times* projected that 2.4 to 24 million people in the United States could require hospitalization, crushing the medical system. The report further emphasized that a worst-case scenario would be 160 million to 214 million people infected in the United States, and projected that the pandemic outbreak could last months or over a year (*The New York Times* 2020, March 13, 2020). Other hypotheticals included schools not being able to open in fall 2020 and pondering how lifting federal restrictions after only thirty days could lead to a drastic spike in cases (Lyons 2020, March 25, 2020).

Last, New York was often mentioned in coverage between March and April 2020, usually with dire outcomes, with reports of the virus "tearing through" New York City and often referencing New York as the epicenter of the virus (Lyons 2020, March 20, 2020). Moreover, on April 3, it was reported that cases rose in New York, with a recorded 100,000 cases and 3,000 deaths. More reports illustrated New York hospitals having trouble getting more health care workers and ventilators to patients who needed them (Takenaga, Tumin and Wolfe, 2020), and on April 6, it was reported that 10,000 people had died in New York because of the virus (Lyons 2020, April 6, 2020).

Mitigation

Early news coverage of the coronavirus in March and April 2020 in *The New York Times* in the United States showed a second main focus was on mitigation, or ways to control the spread of the virus and "flatten the curve" (Lyons 2020, March 11, 2020). On March 9, coverage focused on authorities trying to curtail virus spread rather than fully stop it, since it was infecting individuals at a rapid pace (Lyons 2020, March 9, 2020). Early common mitigation techniques referenced in March 2020 news coverage included social distance mechanisms (usually 6 feet away from others), the cancellation of large "super-spreader" events such as sports, concerts, theatre shows, restricting access to the United States, and asking the public to refrain from traveling and eating in restaurants (Lyons 2020, March 10, 2020). On March 30, it was reported that three in four Americans were under the instruction to stay at home (except for "essential business," such as food shopping, emergencies, etc.). During this same time, *The New York Times* also reported that federal guidelines were being extended another month. These guidelines included previous mitigation techniques such as avoiding nonessential travel, congregating in groups more than ten, eating out and going to work (Lyons 2020, March 30, 2021).

Later mitigation news coverage focused on testing and contact tracing, with much discussion on the importance of testing and unfair access to it, such as famous and wealthy individuals obtaining access before others in the United States. On March 3, it was reported that testing was "ramping up" after weeks of lagging (Lyons 2020, March 3, 2021). On April 16, it was reported that public health officials were urging the use of contact tracing as a prerequisite to reopening the economy and President Trump hoped to begin tracing by May 1, but that it would be an expensive job (Lyons 2020, April 16, 2021). It was also reported that President Trump announced that the CDC would hire hundreds of workers to perform contact tracing and that the federal government would help states pay for their own expanded efforts (Lyons 2020, April 16, 2020). Further, on April 20, reports about disputes over testing availability and strategy in the United States emerged in news coverage, and a discussion of how inadequate testing affected the progress of combating the virus appeared prevalent in *The New York Times* (Lyons 2020, April 20. 2020).

Another mitigation technique mentioned often in *The New York Times* coverage was the use of masks. On March 31, a report was published about the change in mask wearing recommendations. Whereas previously the CDC had said masks should not be worn by the general public, they began suggesting that U.S. citizens wear them in their daily lives (Lyons 2020, March 31, 2020). Similarly, On April 3, *The Times* reported that the CDC began advising all Americans, both healthy and unhealthy, to wear cloth masks when leaving their homes in an effort to slow the pace of the virus. At this time, masks were largely unavailable, even for healthcare workers, and people were finding it difficult to purchase them anywhere. *The Times* also reported that President Trump stressed that the recommendations were voluntary and that he would not be participating in wearing masks (Takenaga, Tumin and Wolfe 2020, April 3, 2020).

A final mitigation subject referenced often in the news coverage of *The New York Times* during March 2020 and April 2020 was pharmaceutical therapeutics. On March 17, it was reported that both drug therapy and the first vaccine studies had begun, and would be expected to take a year at least to complete (Lyons 2020, March 17, 2020). Then on April 27, "a promising vaccine" was reported under development at Oxford University that had potential to be distributed as soon as September 2020 (Lyons 2020, April 27, 2020). Shortly after, on April 29, Lyons (2020) reported on the drug remdesivir and its effectiveness on the COVID-19 virus. Early research suggested that the drug may help people recover faster from the virus, though a competing study suggested it had no effect on extremely ill patients, but *The Times* reported that the FDA was likely to authorize it for emergency use anyhow (Lyons 2020, April 29, 2020). Other drugs mentioned in the same report were hydroxychloroquine, which was described as extremely harmful to use (Lyons 2020, April 29, 2020). According to Lyons (2020) at the time of the report, there were still no approved treatments for COVID-19, though experimental treatments like injecting blood plasma from recovered patients into infected patients was under consideration as a possible remedy for the virus (Lyons 2020, April 29, 2020).

The Economy

A third main focus of news coverage in *The New York Times* during March 2020 and April 2020 was on the economy. On April 2, *The Times* reported that U.S. employers were laying off workers "at an unheard rate" as the virus severely affected the economy (Lyons 2020, April 2, 2020). On March 31, a report mentioned that March was the worst month for Wall Street since 2008, with stocks plummeting to 12.5% on the S&P 500 index (Lyons 2020, March 31, 2020). On April 9, *The Times* reported that 6.6 million people filed for unemployment (Lyons 2020, April 9, 2020), and on April 15 and April 16 they reported that 22 million people had filed (Lyons 2020, April 15–16, 2020), and on April 23, noted that an additional 4.4 million people had filed for unemployment (*The New York Times* 2020, April 23, 2020). Moreover, on April 29, *The New York Times* reported that at the time, the U.S. economy shrank 4.8% which was the biggest rate since the 2008 financial crisis (Lyons 2020, April 29, 2020).

Other news coverage focused on combating the failing economy, with emphasis on stimulus packages designed to help American citizens and businesses. On March 17, *The New York Times* reported that stimulus checks were first proposed in the U.S. government, and on March 20, senators had finalized a 1 trillion-dollar package with direct payments to U.S. citizens (Takenaga, Wolfe and Wright-Piersanti 2020, March 17, 2020). However, on March 23 and March 24 it was reported that no deal could be made for the package between the Democrats and Republicans, but on March 25 it was reported that a new 2 trillion-dollar package was expected to pass through the government quickly (Lyons 2020, March 23-25, 2020). However, on April 15, *The Times* reported that the federal loan program, which was created to help small businesses due to the impacts of the virus, had run out of money (Lyons 2020, April 15, 2020), and then on April 23, a story was published regarding President Trump signing a $484 billion package, which replenished the depleted small-business loan program (*The New York Times* 2020, April 23, 2020).

DISCUSSION

Agenda-setting theory, or the transference of prominent public affairs from the media to the public (McCombs 2005, 543), is apparent in many different arenas, including within political and nonpolitical and cross-cultural spheres (543). First-level and second-level agenda setting thematic analyses indicated that *The New York Times* U.S. COVID-19 coverage during March 2020 and April 2020 revealed three main themes: Dread, mitigation and the economy.

It is not surprising that dread was a major theme in *The New York Times* news coverage during March 2020 and April 2020, and one that they wanted their readers to understand and adopt well. According to Grabe and Kamhawi (2006), "Across time and across media outlets one of the most persistent patterns in journalism content is the high volume and editorial emphasis on negative news" (346). Further, some scholars have suggested that consumers of news actually prefer negative to positive news content and media is simply catering to their news preferences (Trussler and Soroka 2014, 360). This is often referred to as a demand-side rather than a supply side (360), seemingly in opposition to agenda-setting theory. Indeed, studies have found that consumers actually select more negative news content than positive news when given the choice (373). Other studies have described gender differences in consumption of negative news, with males appearing to be enticed by it and women avoiding it, preferring instead to watch more positive forms of news (Grabe and Kamhawi 2006, 346).

Moreover, Shoemaker (1996) believes that journalists feel it is their duty to warn the public against potential survival threats and become watchmen for their communities, serving as a type of surveillance function (36). Historically, during the sixteenth century this process became known as news gathering and the audience appetite for it has remained (Grabe and Kamhawi 2006, 347). According to Grabe and Kamhawi, "this persistent pattern of audience interest in warnings about death, deviance and destruction—or bad news as we have come to call it—bares a cue to our biological wiring" (347). Perhaps, *The New York Times* reported on dread so often because they wanted to drive home and "warn" their readers about the seriousness of the coronavirus pandemic, especially in the early stages of the virus in the United States.

It is also not surprising that mitigation was a prominent theme throughout *The New York Times* news coverage in March 2020 and April 2020. According to the CDC, mitigation is important before a vaccine or therapeutic drug becomes available, especially since COVID-19 is highly transmissible (CDC 2021). In order to lower the risk of infection, the CDC suggests mitigation practices that include healthy hygiene, staying at home when sick, practicing physical distancing, and using cloth coverings (CDC 2021), all techniques mentioned several times in the early stages of *The New York Times* COVID-19 news coverage in the United States.

Further, according to a study by Fuller et al. (2021) European countries that used more stringent mitigation policies had fewer reported COVID-19 associated deaths, suggesting that countries that implemented stricter policies earlier, "might have saved several thousand lives relative to those countries that implemented similar policies, but later" (59). Overall, the research suggests that earlier adoption of mitigation practices (i.e., practicing CDC recommendations in addition to closure of schools, businesses, etc.) may be important in preventing widespread transmission of COVID-19 and decreasing death rates (Fuller et al. 2021, 59).

Because of the importance of mitigation practices in combating the virus, it would make sense then, that *The New York Times* would decide to dedicate a substantial amount of news coverage to information about mitigation techniques, especially during the months of March 2020 and April 2020 when there was a first surge of cases of the virus in the United States.

Last, it is not unexpected that *The New York Times* would commit a significant amount of news coverage to the economy in March 2020 and April 2020. According to Pettinger (2019), a healthy economy thrives on economic growth, and is comprised of higher living standards and incomes, which in turn, allows a society to devote more resources to areas like health care and education. Further, economic growth ensures prosperity (Przeslawska 2016, 137). Additionally, a healthy economy also consists of higher average incomes, lower unemployment, lower government borrowing, improved public services, resources for protecting the environment, encouragement of investments, increased research and development, economic development, and more consumer choices (Pettinger 2019).

When there is an economic threat, like the COVID-19 virus, healthy economies become economies in crisis. According to a report from Bauer et al. (2020, 6), the following economic effects occurred in 2020 as a result of the COVID-19 pandemic: Small-business revenue decreased 20% since January 2020, Chapter 11 bankruptcies increased, decreases in new business formations, declines in total hours worked due to shutdowns and layoffs, and less individuals in the labor force, while the number of unemployed people increased by 4.5 million from January 2020 to April 2020 and has continued to increase. Other findings in the report mentioned that in April 2020 U.S. savings rates reached their highest recorded level, low-income families with children were more likely to experience income shock, in July 2020, one in five households was behind in rent in twenty-six different states, and the rate of food insecurity doubled for households with children (Bauer et al. 2021, 6). Clearly there were several economic impacts caused by COVID-19 in 2020, which is why *The New York Times* may have wanted to focus so much of their news content in this area, especially in the early life of the COVID-19 virus in the United States.

CONCLUSION

The purpose of this chapter was to understand, via thematic analysis, news media coverage in the United States in *The New York Times* during the early months (March 2020 and April 2020) of the COVID-19 virus spread in the United States. Using agenda-setting theory as a framework to guide results, first-level and second-level analyses revealed three prominent themes: dread, mitigation, and the economy. These themes indicate that during the early months of the virus in the United States, *The New York Times* set an agenda about the seriousness and impacts of COVID-19, while also providing information about prevention and protection from the virus. During these two months, they wanted their readers to understand that these topics were of the utmost importance, trumping all other subjects surrounding the pandemic.

LIMITATIONS AND FUTURE DIRECTIONS

Though this research attempted to understand agenda setting within the COVID-19 pandemic, it did not analyze audience reactions to these themes. Future studies should research how these specific themes impacted individual lives and note whether these same topics became salient in the lives of American citizens. Further, future research may also consider analyzing other periodicals to see if similar coverage occurred during related time periods.

REFERENCES

"As Several States Loosen Rules, California Closes Some Beaches." 2020. *The New York Times,* April 30, 2020. https://www.nytimes.com/2020/04/30/us/coronavirus-tracker-live.html?searchResultPosition=13.

Bauer, Lauren, Kristin Broady, Wendy Edelberg, and Jimmy O'Donnell. 2020. "Ten Facts about COVID-19 and the U.S. Economy." *The Hamilton Project,* September 2020: 1–25. https://www.brookings.edu/wp-content/uploads/2020/09/FutureShutdowns_Facts_LO_Final.pdf.

Coleman, Renita, Maxwell McCombs, Donald Shaw, and David Weaver. 2009. "Agenda Setting." In *The Handbook of Journalism Studies,* edited by Karin Wahl-Jorgensen and Thomas Hanitzsch, 147–160. New York: Routledge.

"Coronavirus in the U.S.: 29 Confirmed Cases, More Tests Underway." 2020. *The New York Times,* February 3, 2020. https://www.nytimes.com/2020/02/03/us/coronavirus-united-states-cases.html?searchResultPosition=1.

"Coronavirus Briefing: What Happened Today." 2021. *The New York Times,* March 13, 2021. https://www.nytimes.com/2020/03/13/us/coronavirustoday.html?searchResultPosition=4.

"Death Toll Climbs in California; House Passes Aid Package." 2020. *The New York Times,* April 23, 2020. https://www.nytimes.com/2020/04/23/us/coronavirus-live-news-coverage.html?searchResultPosition=4.

"First Travel-Related Case of 2019 Novel Coronavirus Detected in the United States." 2020. *Centers for Disease Control and Prevention.* January 21, 2020. https://www.cdc.gov/media/releases/2020/p0121-novel-coronavirus-travel-case.html.

Fuller, James A., Avi Hakim, Kerton R. Victory, Kashmira Date, Michael Lynch, Benjamin Dahl, Olga Henao. 2021. "Mitigation Policies and COVID-19-Associated Mortality- 37 European Countries, January 23-June 30, 2020." *Morbidity and Mortality Weekly Report,* 70, no. 2: 58–62. https://www.ncbi.nlm.nih.gov/pmc/articles/PMC7808713/pdf/mm7002e4.pdf.

Gorman, James, and Julian E. Barnes. 2021. "The C.D.C.'s Ex-Director Offers No Evidence in Favoring Speculation that the Coronavirus Originated in a Lab." 2021. *The New York Times,* March 26, 2021. https://www.nytimes.com/2021/03/26/science/redfield-coronavirus-wuhan-lab.html.

Grabe, Maria Elizabeth, and Rasha Kamhawi. 2006. "Hard Wired for Negative News? Gender Differences in Processing Broadcast News." *Communication Research,* 33, no. 5: 346–369. https://doi.org/10.1177/0093650206291479.

Guest, Greg, Kathleen M. MacQueen, and Emily E. Namey. 2011. *Applied Thematic Analysis.* New York: Sage Publications.

"Implementation of Mitigation Strategies for Communities with Local COVID-19 Transmission." 2021. *Centers for Disease Control and Prevention,* February 16,

2021. https://www.cdc.gov/coronavirus/2019-ncov/community/community-mit igation.html#:~:text=Community%20mitigation%20actions%20are%20especially, can%20be%20difficult%20to%20determine.

Lippman, Walter. 1922. *Public Opinion*. New York: Harcourt, Brace and Company.

Lyons, Patrick L. 2020. "Coronavirus Briefing: What Happened Today." 2020. *The New York Times,* March 3, 2021. https://www.nytimes.com/2020/03/03/briefing/c oronavirus-briefing-what-happened-today.html?searchResultPosition=7.

Lyons, Patrick L. 2020. "Coronavirus Briefing: What Happened Today." *The New York Times,* March 9, 2021. https://www.nytimes.com/2020/03/09/us/coronavirus-today.html?searchResultPosition=3.

Lyons, Patrick L. 2020. "Coronavirus Briefing: What Happened Today." *The New York Times,* March 10, 2021. https://www.nytimes.com/2020/03/10/us/coronav irus-today-updates.html?searchResultPosition=4.

Lyons, Patrick L. 2020. "Coronavirus Briefing: What Happened Today." *The New York Times,* March 11, 2021. https://www.nytimes.com/2020/03/11/us/coronav irus-news-today.html?searchResultPosition=5.

Lyons, Patrick L. 2020. "Coronavirus Briefing: What Happened Today." *The New York Times,* March 12, 2021. https://www.nytimes.com/2020/03/12/us/Covid-19 -news.html?searchResultPosition=6.

Lyons, Patrick L. 2020. "Coronavirus Briefing: What Happened Today." *The New York Times,* March 16, 2021. https://www.nytimes.com/2020/03/16/us/coronav irus-today.html?searchResultPosition=8.

Lyons, Patrick L. 2020. "Coronavirus Briefing: What Happened Today." *The New York Times,* March 17, 2021. https://www.nytimes.com/2020/03/17/us/coronav irus-today.html?searchResultPosition=9.

Lyons, Patrick L. 2020. "Coronavirus Briefing: What Happened Today." *The New York Times,* March 18, 2021. https://www.nytimes.com/2020/03/18/us/coronav irus-today.html?searchResultPosition=11.

Lyons, Patrick L. 2020. "Coronavirus Briefing: What Happened Today." *The New York Times,* March 19, 2021. https://www.nytimes.com/2020/03/19/us/coronav irus-today.html?searchResultPosition=13.

Lyons, Patrick L. 2020. "Coronavirus Briefing: What Happened Today." *The New York Times,* March 23, 2021. https://www.nytimes.com/2020/03/23/us/coronav irus-today.html?searchResultPosition=17.

Lyons, Patrick L. 2020. "Coronavirus Briefing: What Happened Today." *The New York Times,* March 24, 2021. https://www.nytimes.com/2020/03/24/us/coronav irus-today.html?searchResultPosition=19.

Lyons, Patrick L. 2020. "Coronavirus Briefing: What Happened Today." *The New York Times,* March 25, 2021. https://www.nytimes.com/2020/03/25/us/coronav irus-today.html?searchResultPosition=20.

Lyons, Patrick L. 2020. "Coronavirus Briefing: What Happened Today." *The New York Times,* March 26, 2021. https://www.nytimes.com/2020/03/26/us/coronav irus-today.html?searchResultPosition=21.

Lyons, Patrick L. 2020. "Coronavirus Briefing: What Happened Today." *The New York Times,* March 30, 2021. https://www.nytimes.com/2020/03/30/us/coronav irus-today.html?searchResultPosition=27.

Lyons, Patrick L. 2020. "Coronavirus Briefing: What Happened Today." *The New York Times,* March 31, 2021. https://www.nytimes.com/2020/03/31/us/coronavirus-today.html?searchResultPosition=28.

Lyons, Patrick L. 2020. "Coronavirus Briefing: What Happened Today." *The New York Times,* April 1, 2021. https://www.nytimes.com/2020/04/01/us/coronavirus-today.html?searchResultPosition=4.

Lyons, Patrick L. 2020. "Coronavirus Briefing: What Happened Today." *The New York Times,* April 2, 2021. https://www.nytimes.com/2020/04/02/us/coronavirus-today.html?searchResultPosition=3.

Lyons, Patrick L. 2020. "Coronavirus Briefing: What Happened Today." *The New York Times,* April 6, 2021. https://www.nytimes.com/2020/04/06/us/coronavirus-today.html?searchResultPosition=7.

Lyons, Patrick L. 2020. "Coronavirus Briefing: What Happened Today." *The New York Times,* April 7, 2021. https://www.nytimes.com/2020/04/07/us/coronavirus-today.html?searchResultPosition=9.

Lyons, Patrick L. 2020. "Coronavirus Briefing: What Happened Today." *The New York Times,* April 8, 2021. https://www.nytimes.com/2020/04/08/us/coronavirus-today.html?searchResultPosition=12.

Lyons, Patrick L. 2020. "Coronavirus Briefing: What Happened Today." *The New York Times,* April 9, 2021. https://www.nytimes.com/2020/04/09/us/coronavirus-today.html?searchResultPosition=13.

Lyons, Patrick L. 2020. "Coronavirus Briefing: What Happened Today." *The New York Times,* April 13, 2021. https://www.nytimes.com/2020/04/13/us/coronavirus-today.html?searchResultPosition=18.

Lyons, Patrick L. 2020. "Coronavirus Briefing: What Happened Today." *The New York Times,* April 14, 2021. https://www.nytimes.com/2020/04/14/us/coronavirus-today.html?searchResultPosition=20.

Lyons, Patrick L. 2020. "Coronavirus Briefing: What Happened Today." *The New York Times,* April 15, 2021. https://www.nytimes.com/2020/04/15/us/coronavirus-today.html?searchResultPosition=21.

Lyons, Patrick L. 2020. "Coronavirus Briefing: What Happened Today." *The New York Times,* April 16, 2021. https://www.nytimes.com/2020/04/16/us/coronavirus-today.html?searchResultPosition=22.

Lyons, Patrick L. 2020. "Coronavirus Briefing: What Happened Today." *The New York Times,* April 20, 2021. https://www.nytimes.com/2020/04/20/us/coronavirus-today.html?searchResultPosition=24.

Lyons, Patrick L. 2020. "Coronavirus Briefing: What Happened Today." *The New York Times,* April 21, 2021. https://www.nytimes.com/2020/04/21/us/coronavirus-today.html?searchResultPosition=25.

Lyons, Patrick L. 2020. "Coronavirus Briefing: What Happened Today." *The New York Times,* April 22, 2021. https://www.nytimes.com/2020/04/22/us/coronavirus-today.html?searchResultPosition=3.

Lyons, Patrick L. 2020. "Coronavirus Briefing: What Happened Today." *The New York Times,* April 23, 2020. https://www.nytimes.com/2020/04/23/us/coronavirus-today.html?searchResultPosition=6.

Lyons, Patrick L. 2020. "Coronavirus Briefing: What Happened Today." *The New York Times,* April 27, 2020. https://www.nytimes.com/2020/04/27/us/coronavirus-today.html?searchResultPosition=9.

Lyons, Patrick L. 2020. "Coronavirus Briefing: What Happened Today." *The New York Times,* April 28, 2020. https://www.nytimes.com/2020/04/28/us/coronavirus-today.html?searchResultPosition=10.

Lyons, Patrick L. 2020. "Coronavirus Briefing: What Happened Today." *The New York Times,* April 29, 2020. https://www.nytimes.com/2020/04/29/us/coronavirus-today.html?searchResultPosition=13.

McCombs, Maxwell E., and Donald L. Shaw. 1972. "The Agenda-Setting Function of Mass Media. *Public Opinion Quarterly,* 36, no. 2: 176–187. https://doi.org/10.1075/asj.1.2.02mcc.

McCombs, Maxwell. 2005. "A Look at Agenda-Setting: Past, Present and Future." *Journalism Studies,* 6, no. 4: 543–557. https://doi.org/10.1080/14616700500250438.

Miles, Matthew B., and Michael Huberman. 1994. *Qualitative Data Analysis (2nd ed.).* Thousand Oaks: Sage Publications.

Nafaria, Ismael. 2018. "The Ranking of the Media with More Pulitzer Prizes." *The New Barcelona Post,* April 17, 2018. https://www.thenewbarcelonapost.com/en/the-ranking-of-the-media-with-more-pulitzer-prizes/.

Pettinger, Tejvan. 2019. "Benefits of Economic Growth." Accessed March 26, 2021. https://www.economicshelp.org/macroeconomics/economic-growth/benefits-growth/#:~:text=The%20benefits%20of%20economic%20growth,a%20rise%20in%20life%20expectancy.

Przesławska Gabriela. 2016. "Rethinking economics in response to current crisis phenomena." *Ekonomia i Prawo. Economics and Law,* 5, no. 1: 133–146. http://dx.doi.org/10.12775/EiP.2016.008.

Salwen, Michael B. 1988. "Effect of Accumulation of Coverage on Issue Salience in Agenda Setting." *Journalism Quarterly,* 65, no. 1: 100–130. https://doi.org/10.1177/107769908806500113.

Shoemaker, Pamela J. 1996. "Hard Wired for News: Using Biological and Cultural Evolution to Explain the Surveillance Function. *Journal of Communication,* 46, no. 3: 32–47. https://doi.org/10.1111/j.1460-2466.1996.tb01487.x.

Taylor, Derrick Bryson. "A Timeline of the Coronavirus Pandemic." *The New York Times,* March 17, 2021. https://www.nytimes.com/article/coronavirus-timeline.html.

Takenaga, Lara, Wolfe, Jonathan, and Tom Wright-Piersanti. 2020. "Coronavirus Briefing: What Happened Today." *The New York Times,* March 20, 2021. https://www.nytimes.com/2020/03/20/us/coronavirus-today.html?searchResultPosition=14.

Takenaga, Lara, and Jonathan Wolfe. 2020. "Coronavirus Briefing: What Happened Today." *The New York Times,* March 27, 2021. https://www.nytimes.com/2020/03/27/us/coronavirus-today.html?searchResultPosition=22.

Takenaga, Lara, Remy Tumin, and Jonathan Wolfe. 2020. "Coronavirus Briefing: What Happened Today." *The New York Times,* April 3, 2021. https://www.nytimes.com/2020/04/03/us/coronavirus-today.html?searchResultPosition=2.

Takenaga, Lara, Jonathan Wolfe, and Carole Landy. 2020. "Coronavirus Briefing: What Happened Today." *The New York Times,* April 17, 2020. https://www.nytimes.com/2020/04/17/us/coronavirus-today.html?searchResultPosition=23.

Takenaga, Lara and Jonathan Wolfe. 2020. "Coronavirus Briefing: What Happened Today." *The New York Times,* April 24, 2020. https://www.nytimes.com/2020/04/24/us/coronavirus-today.html?searchResultPosition=3.

Takenaga, Lara and Jonathan Wolfe. 2020. "Coronavirus Briefing: What Happened Today." *The New York Times,* May 15, 2020. https://www.nytimes.com/2020/05/15/us/coronavirus-today.html?searchResultPosition=27.

Takenaga, Lara and Jonathan Wolfe. 2020. "Coronavirus Briefing: What Happened Today." *The New York Times,* June 11, 2021. https://www.nytimes.com/2020/06/11/us/coronavirus-today.html?searchResultPosition=3.

Trussler, Marc, and Stuart Soroka. 2014. "Consumer Demand for Cynical and Negative News Frames." *The International Journal of Press/Politics,* 19, no. 3: 360–379. https://doi.org/10.1177/1940161214524832.

Wolfe, Jonathan, Lara Takenaga and Tom Wright-Piersanti. 2020. "Coronavirus Briefing: What Happened Today." *The New York Times,* April 10, 2021. https://www.nytimes.com/2020/06/11/us/coronavirus-today.html?searchResultPosition=3.

Wolfe, Jonathan, and Lara Takenaga. 2020. "Coronavirus Briefing: What Happened Today." *The New York Times,* April 24, 2021. https://www.nytimes.com/2020/04/24/us/coronavirus-today.html?searchResultPosition=7.

"WHO Director – General's Opening Remarks at the Media Briefing on COVID-19 – 11 March 2020." 2020. *The World Health Organization,* March 11, 2020. https://www.who.int/director-general/speeches/detail/who-director-general-s-opening-remarks-at-the-media-briefing-on-covid-19---11-march-2020.

"WHO Calls for Further Studies, Data on Origin of SARS-CoV-2 Virus, Reiterates That All Hypothesis Remain Open." 2021. *The World Health Organization,* March 30, 2021. https://www.who.int/news/item/30-03-2021-who-calls-for-further-studies-data-on-origin-of-sars-cov-2-virus-reiterates-that-all-hypotheses-remain-open.

Chapter 5

#Kidstogether

How Nickelodeon Framed Entertainment-Education Messages during the COVID-19 Pandemic

Jobia Keys

The Novel Coronavirus 2019 (COVID-19) pandemic emerged as one of the most dreadful global crises in history, claiming the lives of 1.6 million people as of December 15, 2020 (Roser et al. 2020, par. 1). In addition to the worldwide COVID-19 death toll, there have been over 73 million confirmed cases worldwide (CNN 2020, par. 1), and over 16 million COVID-19 cases and more than 300,000 deaths in the United States (CNN 2020, par. 1).

In the United States, policies were put in place to mitigate and suppress the transmission of COVID-19. Millions of Americans were confined under strict stay-at-home orders and other social distancing measures, such as staying at least six feet away from others and wearing a mask covering the nose and mouth. Reddy and Gupta (2020) note that "fear, distrust, and resistance are common reactions during [a] pandemic," and "trusted and credible information sources are critical for moving people from awareness to action" (3794), thereby emphasizing the important role of public communication during the pandemic.

Because of the ubiquitous nature of COVID-19, parents could not shield their children from the reality of the pandemic. Daily routines were interrupted by school closings, parents working from home, suspended travel, and social distancing measures. Many parents and caregivers sought age-appropriate ways to explain the pandemic, social distancing and stay-at-home orders to their children, and Nickelodeon served as one of many trusted sources for accurate, suitable information about COVID-19.

Ghia et al. (2020) note that children have faced "an overload of information about the COVID-19 outbreak, combining individual concerns, social conversations, mainstream media and social media" (1), and interestingly, "public health information campaigns tailored to children are very rare" (2). Ghia et al. (2020) also argue that cartoons, social media, and appropriate websites are effective tools to "raise awareness among children about the modes of transmission of [COVID-19] [and] the health risks" (3). In addition, researchers note that it is essential for governments, public health experts, education specialists, and media organizations to work together to "meet the needs of children as full-class citizens, whose mental and physical health is as equally important as adults" (Ghia et al. 2020, 3). Nickelodeon gathered a team of trusted medical practitioners and media professionals to help create age-appropriate, informational and entertaining content focusing on COVID-19. Because no previous studies have addressed how COVID-19 health messages are presented to children, this study examined the framing of COVID-19 related messages in select children's programming that aired on Nickelodeon.

In 1979, Nickelodeon premiered as the first American cable television channel for children. During its forty-one-year history, Nickelodeon has been a leader in children's entertainment. While streaming services continue to pull viewers from Nickelodeon and other traditional networks, Nickelodeon is still listed as one of the most-watched networks (Variety 2020, par. 15).

Given that children watch television for entertainment and education, it can be an important means of providing age-appropriate information about COVID-19. This study analyzes Nickelodeon as an entertainment-education source for young viewers to learn about COVID-19. The study also aims to examine Nickelodeon's multiplatform initiative, #KidsTogether, and the strategies and programming used to inform children about COVID-19.

Nielsen (2020) reported an increase in television and streaming viewing among children and teens during the pandemic. In addition to increased television and streaming viewing, many children engaged in virtual learning during the pandemic, and thus spent more time engaging in digital media.

ENTERTAINMENT-EDUCATION

Entertainment-education (E-E) is often implemented as a persuasive strategy within health communication to educate, influence health-related attitudes, and encourage prosocial behavior. Research has supported the effectiveness of E-E messages to increase knowledge about breast cancer (Hether et al.,2008, 820), reduce racial prejudice (Murrar, Sohad, and Markus Brauer 2018, 1075), and prevent the spread of HIV (Schouten et al. 2014, 770).

The E-E approach "has provided a highly effective forum for health education interventions targeting schoolchildren" (Gray et al. 2020, 2). Gray et al. (2020) emphasize that children's televised programming "such as *Sesame Street*... and *Blue's Clues* have contributed to reinforcing positive influences in cognitive development of young children" (2). *Sesame Street's* curriculum and prosocial messages have helped children develop respect and understanding for similarities and differences, get to know people in their community, enhance emotional expression and communication skills, and establish a sense of self (Cole et al. 2018, 67). Mares and Pan (2013) conducted a meta-analysis examining the effects of children's exposure to *Sesame Street* (49). The results of the study indicated an increase in children's literacy, numeracy, world knowledge, social reasoning, attitudes toward out-groups and safety and health knowledge.

Health messages "that are positive, engaging, entertaining, fun and humorous, while providing accurate age appropriate understanding are important features when targeting schoolchildren" (Gray et al. 2020, 2). Effective communication is a vital element in containing a pandemic. Clark, Brudney, and Jang (2013) note that a well-designed communication strategy is a necessity for successful cooperation as a public health response (688). Media play a critical role in disseminating messages to the public, and the messages must be constructed with the particular audience in mind. Given that we are battling a global pandemic, there is an "urgent need to develop specific COVID-19 prevention messages for schoolchildren" (Grey et al. 2020, 2) and Nickelodeon responded to this urgent call with multiplatform E-E programming designed to engage, entertain and educate children about the deadly virus.

Nickelodeon rolled out #KidsTogether in March of 2020. This multiplatform initiative was designed to engage, entertain and inform families. In addition, this global initiative served as an informational resource for families and included short-form videos featuring popular characters, social content, printable activities, and a town hall event (Nickelodeon Press Release 2020, par. 1 and 3).

Nickelodeon's multiplatform initiative is part of ViacomCBS and Ad Council's national campaign to promote healthy habits and encourage unity during the COVID-19 pandemic. This initiative also included a national campaign called #AloneTogether, to educate on the importance of social distancing as a means to prevent the spread of COVID-19. Nickelodeon also used popular characters from their highest-rated shows to share information about COVID-19 prevention. Some of the characters included: *SpongeBob SquarePants, Bubble Guppies, Danger Force, The Casagrandes and Blue's Clues & You* (Nickelodeon Press Release, 2020, par. 5).

COVID-19-RELATED CONTENT ON NICKELODEON

#KidsTogether Town Hall

On March 30, 2020, Nickelodeon aired *#KidsTogether: The Nickelodeon Town Hall*, a virtual hour-long, special program that "directly address[ed] kids' questions and concerns, include[ed] tips and insights from medical experts on ways to be healthy, and [gave] first person accounts from kids and families around the country who [were] social distancing and making changes to their everyday lives" (Nickelodeon Press Release 2020, par. 1).

The #KidsTogether special was simulcast across "Nickelodeon, TeenNick, Nicktoons, and [was] available on Nick On Demand, Nickelodeon, YouTube, the Nick App, and the Nick Pluto TV channel. The special [also appeared] on Nickelodeon's international networks" (Nickelodeon Press Release 2020, par. 4). Actress, Kristen Bell, hosted the town hall event, and special guests joined the show via video conferencing. Guests included medical professionals, celebrities, and music artists.

Short-form Videos

In addition to the town hall event, and as part of the #KidsTogether initiative, original, short-form videos featuring popular characters were created. Nickelodeon aired a series of short-form videos, clips that last five minutes or less. These videos featured popular characters and were embedded in shows, posted on Nickelodeon's social media channels, and aired during commercial breaks. The following Nickelodeon shows featured short-form videos: *SpongeBob Square Pants, Bubble Guppies, Blues Clues & You and Paw Patrol*.

SpongeBob Square Pants

SpongeBob Square Pants is one of Nickelodeon's most renowned animated characters. The *Spongebob Square Pants* show has aired on Nickelodeon since 1999 (Nick and More, 2020), making it the network's longest-running show of all time. The short-form videos that featured SpongeBob Square Pants focused on demonstrating proper handwashing techniques.

Bubble Guppies

Bubble Guppies is an animated preschool television series that has aired on Nickelodeon since 2011 (Nick and More, 2020). The show features mermaid-like characters who go on adventures and speak directly to audiences and convey prosocial messages about responsibility, friendship, healthy habits, and problem-solving. The characters are curious and love to explore. Each episode features songs and stories that promote positive messages. A short-form video featuring the *Bubble Guppies* characters also focused on demonstrating proper handwashing techniques.

Blue's Clues & You

Blue's Clues & You premiered on Nickelodeon in 2019 and is a reboot of the original *Blue's Clues* television series, which originally aired in 1996 (Nick and More, 2020). This is a preschool show that is part live action and part computer animated. The live action character, Josh interacts with Blue, an animated blue dog, to solve problems and puzzles. During the pandemic, this interactive, educational series produced short-form videos that aired on Nickelodeon, YouTube, Instagram, and Facebook.

PAW Patrol

Paw Patrol is an animated series that premiered on Nickelodeon in 2013 to its target audience of preschool-aged children (Nick and More, 2020). The show centers on a young boy named Ryder and a group of six rescue dogs. The crew works together to solve problems and protect their community. Each dog has a special skill that comes in handy during their rescue missions. Nickelodeon released two special, short-form videos during the pandemic to encourage children to wash their hands and stay active and healthy.

Special Episodes

Danger Force

Danger Force is a live action television series that first premiered on Nickelodeon in 2020 (Nick and More, 2020). *Danger Force* is a spin-off series from Nickelodeon's longest-running live action series, *Henry Danger*. The comedy series follows a group of teenage superhero novices who are being trained by their superhero boss as they fight crime in and around their community. Nickelodeon aired a special episode of *Danger Force* with the main characters talking to each other via video conferencing. The episode shows the main characters all hunkering down in their homes during a fictitious quarantine.

The Casagrandes

The Casagrandes is an animated spin-off series from the popular show, *The Loud House*. The show first premiered in 2019 (Nick and More, 2020). Nickelodeon aired a crossover special, "Hangin' At Home," as part of the #KidsTogehter initiative. The short-form video featured the lead characters from *The Loud House* and *The Casagrandes* talking to each other via video conference.

THEORETICAL FRAMEWORK

Reese (2001) defines framing as "the way events and issues are organized and made sense of, especially by media, media professionals, and their audiences" (7). This definition helps to set the premise for understanding how framing can impact audience perception. Framing "approaches provide an excellent theoretical framework for an analysis of media presentations" (Morgan et al. 2007, 144) of COVID-19. Research on health message framing focuses on how the frame of a message impacts its aptitude to encourage healthy behavior.

Media framing analysis has been used to examine a variety of health messages, including but not limited to organ donation (Morgan et al. 2007), fruit and vegetable intake (Elbert & Ots 2018), and vaccine communication (Penta & Băban 2018). Brusse et al. (2017) noted that message framing "has proven to be an effective health communication strategy for promoting behavior change across a wide variety of health behaviors" (1502). Moreover, Ko and Kim (2010) note that "framing messages to match the nature of the issue at hand and to the dispositional tendencies of the target audience can lead people to accept the information, recognize its self-relevance, and encourage behavioral changes" (62). While this study does not focus on behavioral changes, it does, however, analyze how messages are framed within the context of disseminating COVID-19 information.

Media plays a significant role in defining and framing health issues for the public. Media coverage can bring attention to health issues and present causes and solutions for audiences to think about. An important factor that has been "shown to impact the effectiveness of health messages is their framing," and the "specific framing of health messages can increase the effectiveness of [the] messages" (Ko and Kim 2010, 62). This study analyzes the framing of COVID-19 health messages, and it is important to understand how these messages are framed, as they can have a major impact on mitigating the spread of the virus.

METHODOLOGY

Over nine months (March 2020–December 2020), the author watched all COVID-19 related, televised programming that Nickelodeon produced through digital streaming and on-demand cable services. For the purposes of this study, only television programming or video content that aired from March 2020 through December 2020, mentioned COVID-19, social distancing, or proper hygiene was included in this analysis. The following items met the aforementioned criteria:

- *#KidsTogether: The Nickelodeon Town Hall*
- *SpongeBob SquarePants*
- *Bubble Guppies*
- *PAW Patrol*
- *Danger Force*
- *The Casagrandes*
- *Blues Clues & You*

The sample comprised eight short-form videos and three full episodes/specials. A total of eleven media items were analyzed, and each item was coded across a range of factors, including COVID-19 information, social distancing, staying active, and proper hygiene practices.

While this sample does not represent a generalizable sample of all COVID-19 related programming aimed at children, it provides a comprehensive snapshot of the scope of child-centered, televised programming related to COVID-19 and is indicative of public discourse of the pandemic.

The author reviewed each program or short-form video twice. For the initial viewing, the author noted general, recurring frames and coded them accordingly. The author also paid close attention to keywords related to COVID-19 information and prevention and noted the significance of the messaging. For the second viewing, the author noted any additional themes and coded them with the appropriate frames or added new frames if necessary. The author viewed certain scenes and full videos additional times when necessary to better understand and compare frames across programs.

Due to the important nature of the information being disseminated and the vulnerability of the target audience, frames were also examined for alignment with Centers for Disease Control and Prevention (CDC) guidelines. The CDC lists some of the following COVID-19 preventive measures: wear a mask, stay at least six feet away from others who do not live in the home with you, avoid crowds and wash hands often (CDC 2021, par. 1–5).

ANALYSIS

Under the theoretical framework of framing theory, a qualitative analysis of programming was conducted to investigate the presence of dominant frames. Findings revealed that the messages about COVID-19 on Nickelodeon programming fell within four dominant frames: (1) General COVID-19 information, (2) Proper handwashing techniques, (3) Staying active and (4) Social distancing measures.

General COVID-19 Information

The #KidsTogether town hall was the most informative of all programming in the study, and fit well within the "General COVID-19 Information" frame. This 1-hour special included general COVID-19 information, delivered with an audience-centered approach. The information was simple and concise, and included multiple elements to appeal to the target audience of children.

The program featured clips from children all over the country asking questions about COVID-19. Some examples of questions included: Can you play with your friends? How long will it be until we can go back to school? Why is it affecting so many people around the world? Former U.S. surgeon general, Dr. Vivek Murthy, joined the town hall event to answer important questions asked directly by children.

One child asked about the symptoms of COVID-19, and Dr. Murthy explained that "if you have COVID-19, most people have a fever, they can have a cough and most people feel achy, and really, really tired" (Nickelodeon Presents #KidsTogether, 2020). While Dr. Murthy discussed each symptom, cartoon images and clips of characters from Nickelodeon shows experiencing the symptoms appeared on the screen. Dr. Murthy also noted that "COVID-19 seems to spread a lot more easily than the flu, and it seems to be more dangerous as well" (Nickelodeon Presents #KidsTogether, 2020). He further explained to children that the virus spreads when people cough or sneeze and particles from that fluid contain the virus are dispersed. During his explanation, an image of SpongeBob Square Pants coughing and sneezing appeared on a split screen next to Dr. Murthy.

Bell stated, "We've heard a lot of stuff on news and online. And, some of it is true and some of it isn't. And we are going to sort through all of it today" (Nickelodeon Presents #KidsTogether, 2020). Bell introduced a segment called "Fact or Fiction" that focused on debunking common misconceptions about the virus. During this segment, Nickelodeon veterans, Kenan Thompson and Kel Mitchell were asked to determine whether or not each statement was fact or fiction, and Dr. Murthy was there to confirm the validity. For example, one statement read, "the weather will make Coronavirus go away." Both Kenan and Kel guessed that the statement was fiction, and Dr. Murthy confirmed that the statement was fiction. Weather does not affect the virus.

The messages in the town hall special aligned with CDC guidelines. The information emphasized the preventive approach against COVID-19 and reiterated the importance of social distancing, washing hands throughout the day, and wearing a mask in public spaces.

Proper Handwashing Techniques

Demonstrative videos on proper handwashing techniques dominated the short-form video themes. *The SpongeBob Square Pants* video featured the character washing his hands while a voice-over reminds him to clean the front and back of his hands for at least twenty seconds, with a last-minute reminder to clean his knuckles and under his nails. The character is shown washing his hands so vigorously that his hands fall off. While this is clearly an exaggeration of how vigorously one needs to wash their hands, the video aligns with CDC guidelines on handwashing, underscoring the importance of washing the front and back of the hands for at least twenty seconds and washing under the nails (CDC 2021).

A short *Bubble Guppies* video showed the characters demonstrating proper handwashing techniques. The video played during commercial breaks and was posted on the Nickelodeon website and social media channels. This video, however, featured a catchy song called "The Handwashing Song." As the characters dance and sing the song, video clips of real children washing their hands appear next to the animated characters as a visual reminder. One part of the song emphasizes how to properly wash hands by focusing on cleaning the front and back of hands, and the lyrics say, "Gotta use a little soap to wash our hands, get the backs and fronts, yeah that's our plan," and "wash, wash the front of your hands, wash, wash the back of your hands, rub them, scrub them, wash your hands." This video is different from the *SpongeBob SquarePants* video in that it features a song and dance. However, both videos deliver the same information about proper handwashing techniques and align with CDC guidelines.

The *Paw Patrol* video also fit within the "Proper handwashing techniques" frame. This video featured a catchy song, called "Let's Wash up," that emphasized lathering soap and scrubbing both sides of the hands. Unlike the *Bubble Guppies* and *SpongeBob SquarePants* videos, the *Paw Patrol* video did not include images of actual handwashing. Instead, the video included clips from previous episodes of the characters taking baths and playing together. The "Let's Wash up" song focused on proper handwashing from the standpoint of helping to keep others safe and well. The lyrics say, "there's a chance you might get sick, the best gift that you can give to your friends and neighbors to help keep them well is a simple little trick, we just wash our hands like this, so let's keep our hands clean with this routine." This approach emphasizes that one must "wash" and "scrub" hands to get them clean, but it also encourages audiences to wash their hands for the safety of themselves and others.

All three of the short-form videos centered on how to wash hands. This framing worked to position proper handwashing techniques as the common-sense way to prevent the spread of the virus.

Staying Active

Paw Patrol featured a short video with the main characters exercising, to promote physical activity while at home. The exercises included stretches, jumping jacks, dancing, yoga, and running. The video featured a voice-over that encouraged audiences to stand up and exercise, while clips of the characters engaging in the directed exercises played. For example, the voice-over said, "Now it's time for jumping jacks. Follow us!" A clip of one of the characters doing jumping jacks played with a ticking countdown clock in the upper left corner demonstrated how long the audience should engage in each exercise. The CDC recommended engaging in regular exercise during the pandemic to stay healthy (CDC 2021), and this video fit within the "Staying Active" frame and aligned with CDC guidelines.

The #KidsTogether town hall also fit within the "Staying Active" frame. The special featured a celebrity guest appearance by singer, Ciara Wilson and her husband, football star, Russell Wilson. They talked about how they turned their house into an indoor soccer field to have fun with their children at home. Other children chimed in and discussed how they continued to stay active while at home. Some talked about taking walks with their families and others discussed using social media platform, TikTok to learn new dances, have fun and stay active.

Clips of celebrities discussing how they occupied themselves during quarantine were also included in the one-hour special. For example, tennis champion, Serena Williams, showed off her garden and talked about how gardening helped her to stay active and have fun while quarantining. Actor, Anthony Anderson talked about how he exercised and played games with his family, and Actor Ken Jeong, talked about how he stayed active by playing with his new puppy. The celebrities who made an appearance on the special encouraged the audience to "stay strong," "stay safe," and "stay active."

Social Distancing Measures

The virtually produced *Danger Force* special episode, "Quaran-kini" featured the main characters quarantining at home because their fictional town, Swellview, is plagued by a natural gas leak. The gang of superheroes must figure out how to stay busy while in quarantine.

While the episode doesn't specifically mention the words "COVID-19," the entire episode weaves in COVID-19 preventive messaging throughout. For example, the fictional news reporters mirror real-life news reporters, conveying parallel messages about the necessity of social distancing. The reporters, who are seen delivering the news via video conferencing, use key phrases like "shelter in place" and "safer at home" to highlight the importance of staying home when the environment is not safe.

The Casagrandes special episode featured the main characters talking to each other via video conferencing. The characters discussed how they made great use of their time at home. They talked about getting haircuts at home, finding ways to stay busy while under quarantine, celebrating essential workers during the pandemic and making fashionable face masks. The episode also featured clips of classical moments from previous episodes. The special reflected the reality of its target audience depicting the virtual connection between friends during the pandemic. This episode also aligned with CDC guidelines, encouraging people to remain at home, unless necessary and stay at least six feet away from others when out in public.

Blues Clues & You aired short videos, called virtual playdates, and featured Josh interacting with Blue and children who joined via video conferencing. The virtual element of these playdate videos fit within the "Social Distancing Measures" frame. The main characters engage in fun stay-at-home activities like singing, dancing, exercising, and art projects. The videos also featured real children engaging in these "safe-at-home" activities. In addition to encouraging "safe-at-home" activities, the characters demonstrate how to make a dog-shaped peanut butter and jelly sandwich, how to make sock puppets, and encourage the audience to show gratitude for essential workers who help to keep everyone safe.

It is important to note that within the "Social Distancing Measures" frame, there was an emphasis on the importance of spending time with family. Most of the media items in the sample encouraged the audience to spend time with family. The town hall event featured celebrities talking about enjoying family time and medical experts who explained that spending time with loved ones helps to reduce stress during very stressful times. *The Casagrandes* characters talked about spending time with their families, there were also "hanging out family" references in the *Danger Force* special episode. Overall, within the "Social Distancing Measures" frame, spending time with loved ones was consistently encouraged. Also, within the context of the "Social Distancing Measures" frame, social distancing measures were constructed primarily as a collectivist, social practice to prevent the spread of the virus.

DISCUSSION

It is critical to examine the ways in which health-related messages are framed and presented to children because of the potential impact these messages have on children and their families at various levels. This is the first study to analyze frames employed by Nickelodeon to convey important messages about COVID-19.

A sample of short-form videos and special episodes that aired on Nickelodeon was analyzed to identify major frames related to COVID-19 information. This study revealed key findings regarding how messages are constructed for millions of our most vulnerable citizens children. After identifying four key frames across the media content, this framing analysis revealed Nickelodeon's messaging across media items was consistent with professional, COVID-19 related medical information from the CDC. The CDC recommendations that were included in the messaging included: proper handwashing protocol, social distancing, and staying physically active to remain healthy. The study also revealed that Nickelodeon implemented an audience-centered approach with their entertainment-education campaign, focusing on educating audiences about COVID-19 while also keeping them entertained through comedy, music, dance, celebrity guest appearances, and other activities. Children were able to see first-person accounts from other children and families around the country who had to adjust their lives during the pandemic.

Nickelodeon's #KidsTogether campaign content informed audiences about the COVID-19 virus, reinforced good hygiene practices, discussed ways to stay both physically and mentally healthy during the pandemic, and encouraged social distancing. It is possible that the information in the campaign played a key role in enhancing children's and parent's understanding of COVID-19, and may have even helped to mitigate the risk and prevent further spread of the virus. During health emergencies, targeted explanations that help curtail anxiety and fear in young children is important. Nickelodeon's entertainment-education approach was methodically researched, carefully crafted, and followed CDC guidelines for COVID-19 prevention.

LIMITATIONS AND FUTURE RESEARCH

Findings provide evidence of how Nickelodeon might influence its target audience to employ preventive COVID-19 measures by the use of targeted media frames. Longitudinal studies, specifically focusing on the effectiveness of Nickelodeon's entertainment-education campaign, would be beneficial. These future studies could examine whether or not targeted framing has an impact on health-related behaviors. A study of this scope could contribute to the entertainment-education field and help researchers understand the importance of framing in health campaigns as it relates to subsequent health-related behaviors.

In addition, future studies would benefit from examining a broader range of content across multiple children's media channels. For example, analyzing content from PBS Kids, Disney, and Cartoon Network would help broaden our understanding of framing within health campaigns. While this study discussed four central media frames, it is important to note that there may be many other important frames related to COVID-19 information.

CONCLUSION

Message framing has been an essential focus in health communication research. This study revealed that carefully researched, meticulously crafted media frames can add depth to a multiplatform, entertainment-education campaign. This study also expands framing research within an entertainment-education context. In addition, there was no evidence of conflicting COVID-19 related safety precautions or advice, as the findings of this study indicated that Nickelodeon's message framing mirrored CDC COVID-19 guidelines. The content entertained audiences while also educating them about the COVID-19 virus and ways to stay safe and healthy during the pandemic.

REFERENCES

Brusse, Elsbeth D. Asbeek, Marieke L. Fransen, and Edith G. Smit. 2017. "Framing in Entertainment-Education: Effects on Processes of Narrative Persuasion." *Health Communication,* 32 (12): 1501–9. doi:10.1080/10410236.2016.1234536.

Centers for Disease Control and Prevention (CDC). 2021. "Handwashing." Retrieved from: https://www.cdc.gov/coronavirus/2019-ncov/global-COVID-19/handwashing.html.

Centers for Disease Control and Prevention (CDC). 2021. "How to Protect Yourself and others." Retrieved from: https://www.cdc.gov/coronavirus/2019-ncov/prevent-getting-sick/prevention.html.

Clark, Benjamin, Jeffrey L. Brudney, and Sung-Gheel, Jang. 2013. "Coproduction of Government Services and the New Information Technology: Investigating the Distributional Biases." *Public Administration Review,* 73 (5): 687–701.

Cole, Charlotte F., June H. Lee, Abigail Bucuvalas, and Yasemin Sırali. 2018. "Seven Essential Elements for Creating Effective Children's Media to Promote Peacebuilding: Lessons from International Coproductions of Sesame Street and

Other Children's Media Programs." *New Directions for Child & Adolescent Development,* 159: 55–69. doi:10.1002/cad.20229.

Elbert, Sarah P., and Patricia Ots. 2018. "Reading or Listening to a Gain- or Loss-Framed Health Message: Effects of Message Framing and Communication Mode in the Context of Fruit and Vegetable Intake." *Journal of Health Communication,* 23 (6): 573–80. doi:10.1080/10810730.2018.1493059.

Ghia, Jean-Eric, Sophie Gaulin. Laure Ghia L., Laure Garancher, and Claude Flamand C. 2020. "Informing children citizens efficiently to better engage them in the fight against COVID-19 pandemic." *PLoS Neglected Tropical Diseases,* 14 (11): 1–4. https://doi.org/10.1371/journal.pntd.0008828.

Gray, Darren J., Johanna Kurscheid, Mary Lorraine Mationg, Gail M. Williams, Catherine Gordon, Matthew Kelly, Kinley Wangdi, and Donald P. McManus. 2020. "Health-Education to Prevent COVID-19 in Schoolchildren: A Call to Action." *Infectious Diseases of Poverty,* 9 (1): 1–3. doi:10.1186/s40249-020-00695-2.

Hether, Heather. J., Grace C. Huang, Vicki Beck, Shiela T. Murphy, S. T., and Thomas W. Valente. W. 2008. "Entertainment-Education in a Media-Saturated Environment: Examining the Impact of Single and Multiple Exposures to Breast Cancer Storylines on Two Popular Medical Dramas." *Journal of Health Communication,* 13: 808–23. doi:10.1080/10810730802487471.

"Kids and Teens Drive Daytime TV Viewing and Streaming Increases during COVID-19." 2020. Accessed April 1, 2021. https://www.nielsen.com/us/en/insights/article/2020/kids- and-teens-drive-daytime-tv-viewing-and-streaming-increases-during-COVID-19/.

Ko, Deborah M., and Heejung S. Kim. 2010. "Message Framing and Defensive Processing: A Cultural Examination." *Health Communication,* 25 (1): 61–68. doi:10.1080/10410230903473532.

Mares, Marie-Louise, and Zhongdang Pan. 2013. "Effects of Sesame Street: A Meta-Analysis of Children's Learning in 15 Countries." *Journal of Applied Developmental Psychology* 34, no. 3: 140–51. doi:10.1016/j.appdev.2013.01.001.

Max Roser, Hannah Ritchie, Esteban Ortiz-Ospina and Joe Hasell. 2020. "Coronavirus Pandemic (COVID-19)". *Published online at OurWorldInData.org.* December 15, 2020. 'https://ourworldindata.org/coronavirus.'

Morgan, Susan E., Tyler R. Harrison, Lisa Chewning, LaShara Davis, and Mark DiCorcia. 2007. "Entertainment (Mis)Education: The Framing of Organ Donation in Entertainment Television." *Health Communication,* 22 (2): 143–51. doi:10.1080/10410230701454114.

Murrar, Sohad, and Markus Brauer. 2018. "Entertainment-Education Effectively Reduces Prejudice." *Group Processes & Intergroup Relations,* 21 (7): 1053–77. doi:10.1177/1368430216682350.

"Nick and More. List of Every TV Series Aired on Nickelodeon." 2020. Accessed April 1, 2021. https://www.nickandmore.com/kids-tv-history/list-of-every-series-aired-on-nickelodeon/.

"Nickelodeon presents #KidsTogether: The Nickelodeon Town Hall, Hosted By Actress Kristen Bell." 2020. Accessed April 1, 2021. https://www.nick.com/shows/nickelodeon-town-hall.

Nickelodeon Press Release. 2020. Accessed April 1, 20201. https://www.nickpress.com/press-releases/2020/03/27/nickelodeon-presents-kidstogether-the-nickelodeon-town-hall-hosted-by-actress-kristen-bell.

Penţa, Marcela A., and Adriana Băban. 2018. "Message Framing in Vaccine Communication: A Systematic Review of Published Literature." *Health Communication*, 33 (3): 299–314. doi:10.1080/10410236.2016.1266574.

Reddy, Venkatashiva B., and Arti Gupta. 2020. "Importance of Effective Communication during COVID-19 Infodemic." *Journal of Family Medicine & Primary Care*, 9 (8): 3793–96. https://doi.org/10.4103/jfmpc.jfmpc_719_20.

Reese, Stephen. 2001. "Prologue—Framing Public Life: A Bridging Model for Media Research." In *Framing Public Life: Perspectives on Media and Our Understanding of the Social World*, edited by Stephen. D. Reese, Oscar. H. Gandy, and August. E. Grant, 7–31. Mahwah: Lawrence Erlbaum.

Schouten, Barbara, Martijn Vlug-Mahabali, Silvia Hermanns, Esmee Spijker, and Julia van Weert. 2014. "To Be Involved or Not to Be Involved? Using Entertainment-Education in an HIV-Prevention Program for Youngsters." *Health Communication*, 29 (8): 762–72. doi:10.1080/10410236.2013.781938.

"Tracking Coronavirus' Global Spread." 2020. *CNN*, December 15, 2020. https://www.cnn.com/interactive/2020/health/coronavirus-maps-and-cases/.

"Year in Review: Most-Watched Television Networks- Ranking 2020's Winners and Losers." 2020. *Variety*. December 28, 2020. https://variety.com/2020/tv/news/network-ratings-2020-top-channels-fox-news-cnn-msnbc-cbs-1234866801/.

Index

Adams, Tony E., 20
Ad Council, 65
agenda-setting theory, 49–50, 55
#AloneTogether, 65
Anderson, Anthony, 72
Anwar, Ayesha, xiii–xiv
Arbery, Ahmaud, 28
Ashley, Wendy, 29
autoethnography, xiv–xvi, 5–6, 19–20

Bauer, Lauren, on COVID-19 economic impact, 57
Bell, Kristen, 66, 70
Berberoglu, Aysen, 4
Black Lives Matter (BLM) movement, 28
Blue's Clues & You, 65, 69; "safe-at-home" activities in, 73; short-form videos on, 67; social distancing measures frame in, 73. *See also* Nickelodeon
Bochner, Arthur, 5, 20
Bohlen, Stacey, 36
Boyczuk, Alana M., 26
Boylorn, Robin M., 5
Browne, Dillion, 4, 5
Brudney, Jeffrey L., 65
Brusse, Elsbeth D., 68

Bubble Guppies, 65, 69; as animated preschool television series, 66; "The Handwashing Song" featured in, 71; positive messages promotion of, 67; short-form handwashing techniques video on, 67. *See also* Nickelodeon

The Casagrandes, 65, 69; family time in, 73; "Hangin' At Home" crossover special of, 67; time at home use in, 73; video conferencing short-form video of, 68; virtual friend connection in, 73. *See also* Nickelodeon
Caughlin, John P., 13
Center for Disease Control and Prevention (CDC), xiii–xiv, 41, 53; on American Indian and Alaska Native persons pandemic impact, 36; #KidsTogether: The Nickelodeon Town Hall and, 70–71; mitigation practices of, 56; mixed messages and, 3; Nickelodeon guideline alignment with, 69, 71, 72, 74; stay-at-home order and, 49; travel-related COVID-19 detected by, 49
Clark, Benjamin, 65
Clement, J., 39

Coleman, Renita, 50
communication, xiii–xv, 30, 36–37, 40. *See also* in-law communication; interpersonal communication
Communication Theory of Identity (CTI), 20–21
COVID-19 Pandemic. *See specific topics*
Crow Nation, 36
CTI. *See* Communication Theory of Identity

Danger Force, 65, 69; family time in, 73; "Quaran-kini" episode on, 72; social distancing necessity in, 73; video conferencing episode of, 67. *See also* Nickelodeon
data analysis, 39–40, 51
Davis, Denyvetta, 29
Denzin, Norman K., xiv
Dinler, Asim, 4
Dykes, Pamela, xv

economy, 54–57
E-E. *See* entertainment-education
Ellis, Carolyn, 5, 20
entertainment-education (E-E), 74, 75; cognitive development positive influence of, 65; positive health messages and, 65; research on, 64; *Sesame Street* curriculum and, 65
European countries, mitigation practices early adoption of, 56
Expectation Dissonance theory, 42, 44
Expectation Management theory, 43, 44

Facebook, 39, 43, 67
Fletcher, Paula C., 26
Floyd, George, 23, 24, 25, 28
Freberg, Karen, 37
Fuller, James A., 56
Furman University Men's Lacrosse program, 38

Ghia, Jean-Eric, 63–64

Grabe, Maria Elizabeth, 55, 56
Great Depression, 52
Guest, Greg, 51
Gupta, Arti, 63
Guterres, Antonio, 52

handwashing, 41, 66–67, 70–72, 74
"The Handwashing Song," 71
Harris, Kamala, 28
Humphrey, Hubert, 50

in-law communication: autoethnography use in, 5–6; autonomy desire in, 12; Berberoglu and Dinler on family and COVID-19 messages, 4; breakfast outside compromise in, 7–8; close relationship maintaining in, 4; communication style adjustment in, 15; COVID-19 impact on, 5–6; COVID-19 misinformation overload and, 14; COVID-19 research and treatment in, 8; dinner discussion in, 6–7; emotional vulnerability in, 14; face masks and hiking episode in, 8–9; faculty vaccine discussion in, 10–11; family and in-law conversation differences in, 15; family communication style in, 13; family dynamics shift in, 5; in-law vaccine reaction in, 11–12; internal conflict in, 13; marital dyad forming of, 4; mask shaming and, 9; message overload and anxiety in, 3; mindful listening in, 13–14, 16; mother-in-law and mask mandates conversation in, 9; numbers and cause of death discussion in, 6; openness-closedness dialectic negotiation in, 13; peer-reviewed scientific articles confusion in, 14–15; predictability and novelty need in, 12; "preprint" studies and, 15; psychological and interpersonal behavioral processes in, xv; Serewicz on, 4; tension management in, 15–16; triadic structure of, 5 interpersonal communication, xiv; autoethnographical approach in, xv; facial coverings and social distancing in, xiii; intimate communication in, xv; Jones on, xiii

Jang, Sung-Gheel, 65
Jeong, Ken, 72
Johns Hopkins, 3, 6
Jones, Tricia, xiii

Kamhawi, Rasha, 55, 56
Keys, Jobia, xvi
#KidsTogether: The Nickelodeon Town Hall, 69; Bell hosting and video conferencing in, 66; CDC guidelines alignment in, 70–71; celebrity staying active clips on, 72; "Fact or Fiction" segment on, 70; family time in, 73; general COVID-19 information frame in, 70; kids' questions addressed on, 66, 70; Murthy on COVID-19 symptoms in, 70; staying active frame on, 72; as virtual special program, 66. See also Nickelodeon
Kim, Heejung S., 68
Ko, Deborah M., 68
Koerner, Ascan F., xv
Kosloski, Karl, 30

"Let's Wash up" song, 71
Lincoln, Yvonna S., xiv
Lippmann, Walter, 50
Lipscom, Allen E., 29
Loh, Katherine, xv
Lyons, Patrick L., 54

Mackie, Cara T., xv
MacNeil-Kelly, Theresa, xvi
MacQueen, Kathleen M., 51
Mares, Marie-Louise, 65
masks, 8–11, 14, 21, 24, 27, 53–54
mass media: communication changes in, xiii–xiv; information and misinformation on, 4; message communication in, xv; public health issues defining and framing in, xvi. See also The New York Times; Nickelodeon
McCombs, Maxwell E., 50
mental health, xiii, 19, 29
Mikucki-Enyart, Sylvia L., 5, 13
Miller, Dorothy, 25
mindful listening, 13–14, 16
Mitchell, Kel, 70
mitigation techniques, 53–54, 56, 63
Montgomery, Rhonda, 30
Morr Serewicz, Mary Claire, 4, 5
Murthy, Vivek, 70

Namey, Emily E., 51
National Collegiate Athletics Association (NCAA), 38
National Indian Health Board, 36
Native American community, xvi, 38–39; Bohlen on COVID-19 infection rate in, 36; CDC on, 36; COVID-19 impact on, 36, 42; health care and multigenerational living in, 36; Montana statistics for, 36
NCAA. See National Collegiate Athletics Association
Nemo, Leslie, 28
The New York Times: agenda-setting theory use in, 49–50, 55; article selection mandates in, 50–51; COVID-19 thematic analysis of coverage in, xvi, 49–50, 57; criterion sampling use in, 51; data analysis of, 51; dread theme in, 52, 55; economy focus in, 54–55, 56, 57; federal guidelines in, 53; federal loan program report in, 55; first and second level agenda setting in, 50; hypothetical elements focus of, 52; limitations and future directions in, 57–58; March and April 2020 focus of, 51; mask use coverage in, 53–54; media agenda and public adoption

in, 50; medical system projection of, 52; mitigation techniques focus in, 53–54, 56; negative news and gender differences in, 55–56; New York often mentioned in, 52; pandemic and travel bans in, 52; pharmaceutical therapeutics news coverage of, 54; reader warning of, 56; repetitive dire words and phrases in, 52; Shoemaker on journalists duty and, 56; sickness reports in, 52; stimulus packages reports of, 55; testing and contact tracing news coverage of, 53; theme extraction in, 51; three themes in, 51, 55; Trump national emergency declaration in, 52; unemployment rate reports in, 54; Wall Street plunging and event cancellations in, 52; worker layoffs rates in, 54

Nickelodeon, xvi; CDC guideline alignment in, 69, 71, 72, 74; as children's entertainment leader, 64; children television and streaming viewing increase in, 64; COVID-19 health messages framing of, 68; as COVID-19 information source, 63; COVID-19-related content on, 66–68; COVID-19 televised programming on, 68–69; E-E programming of, 65, 74; eleven media items analysis in, 69; four dominant frames in, 69–70, 74; framing definition for, 68; future studies of, 74–75; initial and second viewing frame comparison in, 69; #KidsTogether multiplatform initiative of, 64, 65, 74; media coverage and, 68; media framing analysis use in, 68; medical practitioners and media professionals team for, 64; message framing in, 75; popular character use of, 65; proper handwashing techniques frame on, 71–72; short-form videos on, 66–68, 74; social distancing measures on, 63, 65–66, 69–74; social media and, 64, 66, 71, 72; staying active frame on, 72; ViacomCBS and Ad Council participation with, 65

Nixon, Richard, 50

Obama, Barack, 28
Orbe, Mark P., 5
Oxford University, vaccine development at, 54

Pan, Zhongdang, 65
Paw Patrol, 69; "Let's Wash up" song on, 71; staying active frame and CDC guideline alignment on, 72; washing hands and staying active short-form videos on, 67. *See also* Nickelodeon
Pettinger, Tejvan, on healthy economy, 56–57
Prentice, Carolyn M., 4, 5, 15
Prime, Heather, 4, 5
public information, xvi; children and pandemic reality in, 63–64; COVID-19 death toll and, 63; mitigation policies in, 63; Reddy and Gupta on pandemic reactions in, 63
Public Opinion (Lippmann), 50

quarantine identity: adult children perception in, 27; African American COVID-19 disproportionate rate and, 28; autoethnography research use in, 19–20; Black identity impact in, 27; Black mental health in, 29; cabin fever and quarantine fatigue journal entry in, 23–24; caregiver impact in, 25–27; caregivers and sandwich generation stress in, 26; class session journal entry in, 21–22; COVID-19 back in news journal entry in, 25; COVID-19 mental health impact in, 19; COVID-19 over journal entry in, 24–25; CTI theoretical frame use in,

20–21; Davis on African American women, 29; enacted identity and relational identity conflict in, 30; expectation communication in, 30; father relationship change in, 23, 26; February early rumblings journal entry in, 21; Florida reopening in, 25; Floyd video replay and, 24; "global anti Blackness" and, 19; identity embracing in, 27–28; "identity gaps" notion in, 25; identity layers in, 20; identity negotiation in, 26; ideological shifts experienced during, 19; journal entries analysis in, 20; life normalcy after, 29–30; lonely feeling in, 22–23; make shift classroom in, 22; Montgomery and Kosloski on caregiving and, 30; pandemic and people of color in, 24–25; psychological and emotional and physical impact of, 23; racial identity in, 27–29; racially motivated shootings during, 28–29; racial tensions and, 24; sandwich generation in, 22, 25–26; two crises in, 24; two identity themes in, 25; walls caving in journal entry in, 22–23

Redden, Elizabeth, 14–15
Reddy, Venkatashiva B., 63
Reed, Jaclyn M., 5
Reese, Stephen, 68
Rittenour, Christine, 15

sandwich generation, 22, 25–26
Sesame Street, 65
Shafir, Rebecca Z., 13–14
Shaw, Donald L., 50
Shoemaker, Pamela J., 56
short-form videos, 66–68, 74
social distancing, xiii, 26; Nickelodeon and, 63, 65–66, 69–74; sports diplomacy and, 41, 45
social media: "infodemic" encountered on, 3–4; Nickelodeon and, 64, 66, 71, 72; sports diplomacy and, ix, 37, 38, 44; Thompson, L., and, xv, 39, 42, 43
Soliz, Jordan, 15
SpongeBob SquarePants, 65, 69; CDC guidelines on handwashing in, 71; proper handwashing techniques video on, 66. *See also* Nickelodeon
sports diplomacy: case study analysis for, 39; case study results in, 40–41; as civil institution, 37; COVID-19 and lacrosse in, 38; COVID-19 collegiate sports impact in, 38; Expectation Dissonance and Expectation Management theories use in, 44; "financial Armageddon" in, 38; issues awareness raising of, 43; limitations and future research in, 44; procedure and data analysis in, 39–40; social distancing and, 41, 45; social media themes and, ix, 37, 38, 44; social responsibility in, 42; strategic communication in, 36–37; Tokyo Olympics and World Lacrosse postponements in, 38; Twitter platform use in, 39; virus timeline and, 35. *See also* Thompson, Lyle
sports diplomat: expectations thematic analysis in, 42; role and trust of, 37–38; strategic communicators thematic analysis of, 43–44; Thompson, L., as, 38–39
Stamps, David, 29
stay-at-home order, 3, 49, 63, 73
staying active, 69, 70, 72
strategic communication, 36–37, 43–44

Taylor, Brianna, 28
thematic analysis, xvi, 42–44, 49–50, 57
Thompson, Kenan, 70
Thompson, Lyle: case study analysis of, xvi, 38; communication focus of, 40; COVID-19 interviews of, 41; COVID-19 related content and, 39–40; COVID-19 video message

of, 40–41, 44–45; diplomatic responsibilities of, 43; Expectation Dissonance theory and, 42; fan base presence of, 43; as lacrosse and Native American community sports diplomat, 38–39; no backlash against, 42; posting amount by, 42; social media and, xv, 39, 42, 43; Tweet subjects of, 43; Twitter activity summary of, *40*; Twitter feed tracking and articles about, 39–40; younger generation addressing of, 41

Tinker, T., 37
Tokyo Olympics, 38
Trump, Donald, 52, 53, 54, 55
Twitter, 39–44

vaccine, 10–12, 54
Vaughan, E., 37
ViacomCBS, 65

video conferencing, 66, 67, 68

Wade, Mark, 4, 5
Wagner, P., 20
Wall Street, 52, 54
WHO. *See* World Health Organization
Wilkes, Sybil, 28
Williams, Serena, 72
Wilson, Ciara, 72
Wilson, Russell, 72
World Health Organization (WHO), 52; COVID-19 and, xiii; COVID-19 progression tracking of, 35; mixed messages and, 3; virus origin investigation of, 49
World Lacrosse, 38
Wuhan, China, xiii; COVID-19 genesis in, 49; as "viral pneumonia" case in, 35

YouTube, 43, 66, 67

About the Authors

Dr. Theresa MacNeil-Kelly is an assistant professor of Communication at Florida Southern College. She has researched many different topics in interpersonal communication, including how people manage conflict in specific contexts such as friendships, families, romantic relationships, and in work environments. She loves learning, researching, and teaching others about communication because it is an area that all types of people can learn and apply to their own lives. Dr. MacNeil is also a Florida State Certified Mediator in family mediation. She started mediating in 2012 for the Connecticut Human Rights Organization and has received three different certifications in mediation training. Her experience and expertise has helped many people resolve their differences.

Dr. Pamela Dykes has successfully made a major impact in the lives of hundreds of individuals in organizations through her work in management, training and development, consulting, coaching, and teaching. She has worked for companies such as Accenture Consulting, and Allstate Insurance Company. Currently she is an Assistant Professor at Florida Southern University. She has also taught at several universities including Denison, Capital, Ohio University and the Ohio State University. Dr. Dykes earned her PhD in Organizational Communication and is a Master Certified Christian Coach. She is also a member of The International Coach Federation, International Christian Coaching Alliance, and the Tampa Bay Professional Coaches Association.

Dr. Jobia Keys is an author, educator, and communication expert who specializes in helping business professionals and organizations embrace diversity and inclusion. She is passionate about cultivating the inclusion, representation, and advancement of diverse individuals in the workplace, and supports inclusion initiatives from evaluations to recommendations to implementation. Her research focuses on cultural studies, gender, race and class representations across all media channels, entertainment-education, media literacy, children's health education, interpersonal communication and intercultural communication. She has presented her work at schools, special events, and national and international academic conferences. She earned her PhD in Communication from the Georgia State University.

Dr. Katherine Loh is an assistant professor in the Communication Department of Florida Southern College, teaching Fundamentals of Speech, Intercultural Communication and Persuasion. Dr. Loh serves as the Lambda Pi Eta advisor (Communication honor society). She is also the NCAA Faculty Athletic Advisor for Florida Southern College. She has been teaching at Florida Southern College since 2010. Dr. Loh has more than twenty years of teaching experience. She has taught at the College of Notre Dame of Maryland, Towson University, and Polk State College. She was also the senior consultant overseeing the Faculty and Staff Development Program at the University of Pittsburgh. Outside of academia, Dr. Loh is the secretary general of the Pan-American Lacrosse Association. She serves on the board of Peru Lacrosse Association and was on the team that successfully took Peru's first Men's National Team to the 2018 World Lacrosse Championship. She also serves on World Lacrosse's Nominating Committee.

Dr. Cara T. Mackie is an associate professor and chair of the Department of Communication at Florida Southern College. Her research focuses on how illness shapes one's identity in turn affecting interpersonal relationships and networks. Her previous work focused on substance abuse, eating disorders, and women and gender studies. She explores critical qualitative research methods and writing, including auto/ethnography, performance inquiry, and narrative.

www.ingramcontent.com/pod-product-compliance
Lightning Source LLC
Chambersburg PA
CBHW020130010526
44115CB00008B/1053